OPTIMAL LIVING WITH YOGA

Ten minutes of Yoga practiced in the morning (starting out while still in bed!) sets an exhilarating mental and emotional tone for the entire day. Ten minutes of Yoga before going to bed improves skin tone and hair luster, creates a suppler, healthier body, and prepares the way for deep, restful sleep.

In **Yoga for Personal Living,** Richard L. Hittleman has created a practical guide for everyone—office worker, housewife or student—who wants to reap the benefits of Yoga in better health, better looks, less tension, more vitality.

D1264664

Other Paperback Library Books
by Richard L. Hittleman

Be Young With Yoga
Yoga For Physical Fitness

For information on ordering the above books, please turn to the last page.

YOGA FOR
PERSONAL LIVING

RICHARD L. HITTLEMAN
YOGA
FOR PERSONAL LIVING

**WARNER
PAPERBACK
LIBRARY**

A Warner Communications Company

WARNER PAPERBACK LIBRARY EDITION

First Printing: May, 1972
Second Printing: August, 1974

Cover photo from Yoga for Health television series

Warner Paperback Library is a division of Warner Books, Inc.,
75 Rockefeller Plaza, New York, N.Y. 10019.

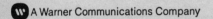 A Warner Communications Company

Printed in the United States of America

To Joshua—an old Yogi in a new body

ACKNOWLEDGMENT

The author wishes to acknowledge the valuable assistance of Lore Kuhns, Yoga for Health instructor in Carmel, California, in the preparation of this work.

CONTENTS

Cover and inside photographs by Stan Bruns, Carmel

YOGA FOR
PERSONAL LIVING

INTRODUCTION

"How much time will I need to devote each day to learn Yoga?" This question is inevitably asked of me within the first five minutes of conversation with a prospective student. Time is a major consideration; time is limited, budgeted, jealously guarded. If this same question were asked of a guru in India, his response would be, "If you have to ask about time you are not yet ready to practice Yoga." This reply is based, understandably, on the ancient tradition of *total involvement* in the study. But as a Yoga teacher who has instructed Americans and Europeans for twenty years and who is well aware that to them time is indeed of the essence, my answer is, "As little time as you wish; ten minutes a day is adequate!" And this answer is quite true. It is possible to practice Yoga on a very limited basis, as tens of thousands of people are currently doing, and still experience highly significant benefits. Of course, I know from a good deal of experience that as soon as the great effectiveness of Yoga is realized, the original ten minutes with which many people begin usually stretch into twenty and twenty, not infrequently, become forty and more. In other words, as Yoga becomes more and more meaningful, additional time is miraculously found for its practice. This is why I encourage people who are interested in Yoga to go ahead with it even though they feel they will have minimal time to spend. Indeed, if you will spend ten minutes each day with one or more of the suggestions offered in this book, you will actually be utilizing an effective amount of Yoga in your daily life.

1

The busier you are the more you may need some Yoga. In my classes I have had the opportunity to show some of the busiest, most active people in our society that the remarkable Yoga science is a completely practical method to achieve health and beauty for the body and peace for the mind and spirit. This wonderful *practicality* of Yoga is the underlying theme of all my teachings. In previous writings I have dealt with the practical application of Yoga in specific areas: physical fitness, body and figure development, weight control, philosophy and meditation, and nutrition. This book contains a total perspective of practical Yoga through the application of all of these aspects. Here I have drawn upon my personal experiences as well as those of my students to illustrate the many ways in which Yoga exercises, breathing, hygiene, nutrition, philosophy, and meditation may be *directly incorporated into the activities of daily life,* on what is almost an around-the-clock basis. As you read through these pages, you will learn how people who are involved in many of the same daily activities and who must confront the same daily situations as yourself are using Yogic principles to deal effectively with certain problems and to aid in the general enrichment of their lives. These principles make good sense. They are the distillation of many centuries of wisdom and are as pertinent today as they were when used a hundred or a thousand years ago. In the next day or two try a few of the things that are suggested. You don't have to undertake everything; simply select what attracts you and let the rest go for later. You will be surprised at how quickly you get the "feel" of the various techniques and at how really helpful they are. You will certainly benefit in an immediate way from whatever you choose to do; frequently the results are dramatic. But perhaps most important of all, is that you may find even a little serious application of Yoga begins to add a new and extremely meaningful dimension to your life.

Richard Hittleman
Carmel, California

ARISING
(a 10 minute routine)

We spend our sleeping hours, at least one-third of our lives, in a state so deep, so profound and mysterious that we have no knowledge of an "identity" and no thoughts of being involved in any other mode of existence. Yet during our waking hours we feel that *this* is our real life and the most we can occasionally remember about our sleeping state is a few moments of dreams. This phenomenon has led Yogic gurus (as well as Zen masters) to pose certain riddles to their students: "Where is your 'identity' when you are asleep?" "Which condition is closer to your true 'self,' waking or sleeping?" Such questions are intended to make the student examine an area of his life that he usually comes to take very much for granted, and reflection upon these questions sometimes produces a fascinating type of "awakening," quite different from the one we experience each morning. But more of this later.

These two states, waking and sleeping, alternating with such daily regularity, are obviously interdependent: our being awake eventually requires us to sleep, and sleep, with its magical powers of renewal, prepares us for our waking hours. As far as we can perceive, we pass into and remain in the sleeping state without conscious effort; usually, no special techniques are needed. But the waking hours require, in addition to just normal activity, the application of many special techniques, not only to cope with the various complex situations in which we continually find ourselves but in order to grow, evolve, achieve some degree of fulfillment in our lives. Because the special techniques with which we are concerned in Yoga profoundly influence one's mood, because they can set the "tone" for the entire day, the routine of physical and mental exercises in this chapter is highly recommended upon re-entering the waking state.

There is another and equally important area in which this routine can be used to great advantage: when a child awakens he is filled with joy in anticipation of the new day. Not many adults awaken with this joy. Because of the peculiar machinelike qualities that the mind acquires as we grow out of childhood, a *continuum* is established: the moment we awaken we tend to effect a connection with our previous waking hours. We make an intensive effort, usually unconsciously, to recall instantaneously our identity, where we are, and the activities in which we are currently involved. Almost simultaneously we take our mental and emotional pulse to determine how we are feeling about these activities and about the world in general. If the sum total of our current activities appears to represent a "gain," if today our balance sheet is on the "plus" side, we will probably tend to react positively toward awakening; life is tolerable—not joyous as with the child, but more than bearable. Conversely, those mornings in which we find ourselves in the "loss" column, life is questionable and getting out of bed difficult, perhaps even painful. As stated, these connections and evaluations are made almost instantaneously upon awakening so that we create an immediate and permanent continuity in the waking part of our life, each morning connected as quickly as possible to the previous evening. Reverting to the child for a moment: his joy in the new day is due largely to *a weakness or break in this continuity*. Upon awakening, his connection is made with the immediate presence of the world, simply with the sense of his existence rather than with his identity, with yesterday. His mind, being relatively free, unfettered, permits him to become acutely aware of an aspect of life that has been largely lost to us, and he rejoices in feeling and responding to it in a very immediate manner. This joy, however, need not be confined to the child. It results directly from the way in which one perceives the world and is absolutely not contingent on age or, indeed, on any external circumstance. It is both possible and important to regain this youthful sense of joy and wonder when we awaken, but in order to do so it is necessary that *we temporarily forget ourselves, that we interrupt our continuity of identity, our connection to yesterday by at least delaying the familiar cycle of thoughts that sweeps us back mentally into all of the domestic, business, and social activities in which we are currently involved.* In place of these thoughts I am suggesting that we substitute a few minutes of mental and physical exercises that will allow us to become aware of our selves in a totally different way, akin to that which the child experiences. This new awareness, even though of momentary duration in the beginning, is of the greatest possible significance in Yoga.

Let me summarize what we intend to accomplish with our "arising" exercises:

1. Become aware of the miracle of being alive and experience the joy that accompanies such awareness.
2. Set an exhilarating mental and emotional "tone" for the entire day.
3. Help prepare the body to function at its optimum level for whatever activities are necessary.

OBSERVATION OF THE BREATH
(1 minute)

This exercise is done the moment your waking consciousness begins to function. You remain in bed in whatever sleeping position you find yourself and with your eyes still closed *simply observe your breathing for approximately one minute.* All you need do is feel, become aware of how you are breathing. However, the thoughts that establish your "identity" and connect you with yesterday tend to flow into your mind with such rapidity once you are awake that in the beginning it is necessary to be very much on guard. Remember, the point is to *delay* these thoughts, to short-circuit the computer, to interrupt the continuity. After a few mornings you will have established the habit of observing your breathing immediately upon awakening, but at first you have to make the very worthwhile effort of preventing these thoughts from carrying you away both before you begin and during the exercise. Upon first reading this, you may think that it is improbable that during the course of only one minute you can be swept away many times by thoughts against your desire, but the power of the computerized, programmed mind is extremely great.

Let me indicate here, with approximate wording, the way in which I learned this exercise. These words may prove helpful; they indicate how the mind can be trained on the exercise.

I have returned from sleep to the "conscious" state. . . . I am aware at this moment that I am awake. . . . it does not matter now who I am or what I must do today. . . . I will think about that later . . . but now my mind will remain free of any thoughts except those that pertain directly to my breathing. . . . I will lie here quietly with my eyes closed, turn my full attention into myself, and become aware of my life, my breathing. . . . I won't force or regulate the breath, I'll continue to breathe exactly as I now am and simply observe the process . . . (and you begin . . . inhalation . . . exhalation . . . inhalation . . . exhalation . . . *here is a thought attempting to distract me; I will dismiss it until later.* . . . (inhalation . . . exhalation . . . etc.).

Naturally you are not to time this one minute exercise with a watch. You will find you are breathing from nine to fifteen times per minute in your lying position so you can either judge the length of one minute or count to the maximum of fifteen, but do not let the counting become automatic while your mind wanders elsewhere. The essential thing is to remain aware of and be fully in touch with the miraculous function of breathing. Your mind, your entire being merges with and *becomes* the breathing.

PREPARING FOR THE MOVEMENTS

When Observation of the Breath is completed you should arise slowly (never jump out of bed, it's not good for the heart or the nervous system) and attend to the elimination needs of the body. As soon thereafter as possible, before washing, shaving, or any other activity that will encourage your mind to fill with thoughts and promote your "identity," the exercise routine of this section should be performed. (Incidentally, it may be necessary for you to awaken approximately ten minutes earlier than has been your custom so that you can complete this routine quietly and privately. Remaining undistracted is essential.)

Minimal clothing or any loose-fitting sleeping attire is satisfactory dress for the exercises; you must have freedom to stretch your arms and legs in all directions. If you are going to change into exercise clothing, don't take too long to do it. We want to begin the exercises as shortly as possible after arising to maintain the mood of introversion we have established with the Observation of the Breath. Make sure there is an open window in your practice area. You must have an abundant supply of fresh air during the performance of these exercises. If your circumstances permit you to be outdoors for the brief practice session, this is ideal.

Obtain a mat or large towel to lay on top of your practice surface. Select this mat carefully; certain bright or "loud" colors and their combinations can emit vibrations that disturb the emotional body, so choose something with subdued, darker tones that are pleasing to your eye. I recall conducting a short seminar in which a highly enthusiastic, elderly lady appeared with an enormous beach towel. On it was written, in shrieking green and orange letters, "HAVE A HAPPY DAY." The towel was extremely disturbing, but because the lady was so delightful and there were to be only three classes, I decided not to dampen her spirits and simply averted my eyes from her direction as much as possible. At the close of the final class she came to me, told me how much she enjoyed the seminar, and, as a token of her appreciation, presented me with her towel!

Put away your mat carefully after practice and do not use it for anything else. This mat will gradually accumulate positive vibrations and eventually these will be transmitted to you by simply sitting or lying upon it.

An easily read watch or clock may prove helpful to establish a time feeling for the various exercises.

Finally, I always suggest a medical checkup before beginning any physical program.

PRANAYAMA (YOGIC BREATHING)

"You can have all the energy and life force you need; just learn how to breathe!" I was nine years old when this was told to me by the first person I had ever seen practicing Yoga. He was a middle-aged Hindu from Malabar, India, who worked as a handyman for my parents and whom I knew as "James." One afternoon I was playing in a secluded wooded area near our place of business in upstate New York when I was attracted to a small clearing by a peculiar hissing sound. There I saw James seated in a Lotus position upon a flat rock. His eyes were closed and he was performing an intensive series of inhalations and exhalations. Although I had known him for some time and felt very close to him, I was startled at his appearance. Whatever he was doing had transformed his face, his entire presence. He was withdrawn, unaware of me or, it seemed, of anything in this world. It was the first time I had ever seen anyone withdrawn in this way, disengaged from the life around him, functioning on another plane. I remember how I stared at him, utterly fascinated, sensing something urgent about what he was doing. He continued his unworldly breathing for some time, eventually stopped, and then remained completely motionless. Now his stillness was so intense it was as though he had turned to stone. I can remember deciding he had stopped breathing altogether and was dead. Even so, I remained transfixed and entertained no thoughts

8

about leaving the scene and bringing help. After what seemed like an eternity but was probably no more than two or three minutes, he opened his eyes, turned his head, and looked in my direction as if he knew all along that I was there. I knew I had intruded upon something very private and I felt embarrassed. But he registered no emotion, no anger, no surprise. He extended the same cordial greeting he always gave me and motioned for me to come and sit near him. It was no use pretending I hadn't seen what he was doing, and I was so relieved that he wasn't dead that I simply asked him outright what it was all about. His reply, which turned into a lengthy explanation, filled me with a great wonder. In his quiet, mellifluous Indian voice he told me things that afternoon concerning the structure of the body and the nature of the mind that completely changed the way in which I saw the world and that I have never forgotten.

He was, of course, practicing a Yoga breathing exercise. He had studied Yoga for a short time first as a child and later in an Indian *ashram,* and he related to me the things that he had learned and experienced there. He had continued his practice wherever fortune had taken him and even now did his exercises each afternoon. Soon I was joining him in these sessions; that was my introduction to Yoga. (Incidentally, at his suggestion it was several years before I spoke to anyone regarding my interest in Yoga. The word "Yoga" in 1936 America was, for the most part, associated with *Terry and the Pirates, Little Orphan Annie's* friend Punjab, and the evil Oriental villains in the Saturday afternoon movie serials.) But the thing James told me that afternoon that fascinated me most, and that I still vividly recall, had to do with the breath. He described the nature of *prana,* the life force that is in the air; he told me it sustains our lives and *how we can change our lives by changing our breathing!* Although I have now been practicing Yoga breathing routines for thirty-five years, I have never ceased to be astonished at their effectiveness, at how each is able to accomplish exactly what it is designed for.

Tired? Run down? Headaches? Tense, nervous, easily upset? Poor circulation? You can get help from an end-

9

less number of products at your local pharmacy. But for many centuries before Madison Avenue made these conditions universally popular and socially acceptable, Yogis were practicing various exercises and methods of breathing to help prevent or remedy such afflictions in a completely natural manner. It does seem incredible that the way in which we breathe can have such a profound effect on our health, our emotions, and our minds, but such, indeed, is the case. And the Yogic breathing methodology goes even further: there are techniques that help us to awaken and use very powerful forces that lie dormant, asleep within us; forces that most of us never even suspect we possess. I must add that James had a beautiful, poetic style of speech, and this certainly lent a touch of romance and fantasy to the whole business—something to which a youngster might be highly susceptible. But in later years when I seriously undertook the study of *Kundalini* Yoga, which deals with the methodical arousal of the "sleeping energy," whatever doubts or notions of fantasy I may have retained were soon dispelled in the light of the profound experiences that are induced by this study.

On the following pages I offer a combination of two breathing exercises that I have found extremely practical and immediately effective. In essence, I present them in a form only slightly modified from that which was taught to me many years ago. When we awoke—a few minutes ago—we simply observed our breathing; we made no effort to change or interfere with its rhythm. But in preparing for the activities of the day, we want to energize our bodies and make our minds alert. Therefore, we *will* now regulate our breathing in two distinct ways: a very quick, forceful breath pattern, followed by a deep, slow one. In connection with these I repeat to you what was told to me one afternoon thirty-five years ago, "You can have all the energy and life force you need. Just learn how to breathe!"

CHARGING—COMPLETE BREATH
(2 minutes)

Traditionally, Yogis face the east during their morning exercise routines to greet the new day and to receive powerful vibrations of energy emitted from the rising sun. I suggest you also face east, even though you live in a megalopolis apartment house, snow is falling, and a compass may be necessary to determine the proper direction.

Our objective in the Charging Breath is to invigorate ourselves, to literally "charge" the body with *prana,* life force, through a series of quick, forceful, sharp inhalations and exhalations. The effectiveness of these movements is dependent on your ability to distend or push your abdomen out during the inhalation, and to contract, pull in forcefully for the exhalation. You're going to have to practice these movements a few times before you catch on to the knack of *pushing out with your stomach as you inhale.* This movement requires extra attention because almost without exception the various systems of calisthenics that you may have done previously required you to take a so-called "deep breath" by pulling your abdomen and diaphragm in and up toward your chest. (Just think for a moment of your movements when the instructor exhorted, "Now take a deep breath.") But in so doing you actually prevent a really deep or what we call "complete" breath from occurring because the lower part of the lungs are cut off through this contraction of the abdomen. To effectively fill the lower part of the lungs, which is our concern in this exercise, the abdomen must be pushed out with your abdominal muscles while you simultaneously inhale. This is actually a much more natural and, in my experience, more healthful way to inhale, and you can observe such breathing in infants and youngsters. Professional singers are well trained in "diaphragmatic" breathing. If you follow the inhalation as described above, the exhalation will be automatic. Your abdomen will naturally contract as you exhale; however, because we want to make this a very forceful expulsion of the air, we utilize the abdominal muscles to intensify the contraction: we pull in quickly and deeply so that the air is "shot" through the lungs and out the nostrils (all breathing in these routines is done through the nostrils).

Now let's try the movements and don't be discouraged if success is not immediate. During the learning period you will notice significant benefits from even the most modified form of this breathing. Incidentally, the forceful inhalations and exhalations will be noisy; this is natural and is encouraged especially in the initial learning stages. If you are not making a fair amount of noise with your nostrils, you will not derive the full benefits, so don't be afraid to let go and "snort." If there is someone asleep in your practice area, you'll simply have to hope for the best. (One of my students induced his wife, who did not share his enthusiasm for the morning Yoga routine, to wear ear plugs to bed.)

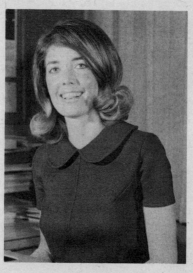

Sally Parodi is a wife and mother of two children. She has been practicing Yoga for one year, during which time she has lost 30 pounds. However, it is the philosophic implications of the Yoga practice that have become particularly meaningful in her life.

FIG. 1

Stand erect but relaxed on your mat. Forget about breathing for a moment and simply work your abdominal muscles, attempting to distend your abdomen, that is, to make a big belly.

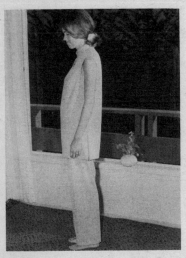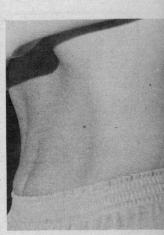

FIG. 2

Quickly, suddenly, forcefully contract your abdomen as deeply as possible. Repeat the movements: distend as far as possible; contract quickly and forcefully, pulling the abdomen in as far as possible. Practice a few times to gain some control. Do the best you can today. The muscles will learn and tomorrow you will note the improvement. Now let's incorporate the breathing. As you push out the abdomen as in Fig. 1, *simultaneously* inhale through your nose. Pause one second. Now contract quickly, forcefully, deeply and assist your lungs in "shooting" the air out sharply through your nostrils.

Repeat: inhale and distend—pause momentarily; contract and exhale—pause momentarily. Practice to make the inhalations and exhalations sharp and rhythmic, pausing just momentarily at both ends. <u>Repeat 10 times.</u>

Frequent complaint from beginning student: "My nose is all 'stopped up' in the morning and it's difficult for me to breathe through it." *Answer: Do your best. Take in whatever air is possible and if you cannot do ten rounds, then do five or even three; rest a moment and try again. This exercise will actually help to open your nostrils and aid the congested condition. If your nose is all 'stopped up,' you may have a structural problem in which case you should consult your physician or examine your living habits. Perhaps the smog has become so bad in your city that you had better consider moving; perhaps your diet needs a radical change; perhaps your general breathing habits should be altered. Many of my students who gasped and wheezed their way into our beginning class experienced a remarkable improvement in their noses and lungs by performing the breathing exercises seriously and following the Yogic nutrition suggestions.*

Following the 10 Charging Breaths we performed above, we execute the exact opposite type of breath—a long, slow, quiet one. This is the "Complete Breath."

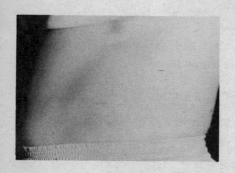

FIG. 3

Upon completion of the tenth Charging Breath, pause a moment and then begin a very deep, very slow inhalation. As you inhale distend your abdomen exactly as you did previously (only now very slowly) so that the air may enter the lower area of your lungs.

14

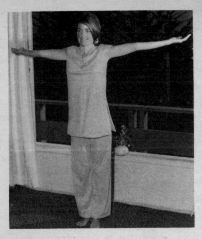
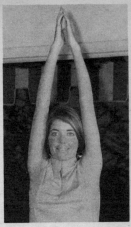

FIG. 4

Continue the deep, slow inhalation. Start to expand your chest and simultaneously raise your arms as illustrated. This must all be done very slowly.

FIG. 5

Continue the same deep, slow inhalation (you can see it will have to be a slow and deep one or at this point you will have run out of inhalation before you have completed the necessary movements). Now expand your chest fully (your abdomen will automatically contract) and have your palms meet overhead. This raised position of the arms permits the air to enter the high area of your lungs.

Retain the air for a count of 5.

Very slowly exhale, simultaneously bringing your arms very slowly back to your sides. (Control the exhalation; don't allow the air to rush out.)

Pause without moving for a few moments and begin the next round of 10 Charging Breaths followed by 1 Complete Breath. Perform the entire routine 5 times in all. When perfected, 5 times will require 2 minutes.

Note: The Complete Breath will help remedy shallow breathing and short-windedness. It fills your lungs with air more completely, gently, and methodically than any breathing exercise I know of.

ABOUT LIFE FORCE

When you have been involved with Yoga for a while, your view of your body begins to change. You come to feel it less in physical terms, that is, as a dense structure with bones, muscles, organs, and so forth, and more in etheric or spiritual terms, as a manifestation of cosmic thought. You remain very much aware of the body; indeed, the nature of the Yoga exercises allows you to become more profoundly "in touch" with it than ever before. But because these exercises fill your organism with an unprecedented lightness and vitality, a refinement takes place; you gradually transcend the lower, gross planes of existence and ascend to a higher plane. There, your new awareness of all things, the physical body included, occurs from the vantage point of an expanded consciousness. Certain *subtle* elements of existence, which you may have seen and felt darkly or understood abstractly, are now more clearly perceived and more directly experienced. Such concepts as love, compassion, charity are no longer words with mundane associations but are ever-present *realities*. These things are now known to you in more absolute terms because you have achieved a major goal of Yoga, that is, a union or merger with the dimensions where truth is not filtered through the senses and intellect but where it is *directly experienced*.

One of the most revealing of these perceptions is in regard to life force. You come to recognize more and more the presence of this subtle element that the Yogis have explained in such great detail as being the substance that sustains life. And as your sensitivity to its nature grows, you can begin to evaluate the states of your physical and emotional health in terms of life force. You will know that you must be receiving and retaining a sufficient amount of life force to function at your optimum; if your life force falls below what is the proper level for you, your health and activities will suffer proportionately. There is no guesswork on your part regarding this, and no external authority will need to tell you about your life force. You will know without the slightest doubt whatsoever when your life force is below par and you will be able to take steps to increase it. This is very much in keeping with the "self-reliance" concept of Yoga, which teaches turning more and more into oneself to seek the solutions for certain problems.

The major sources of life force that pertain directly to our physical organism are air, sleep, water, food, and light (sun). There are others, less important, that need not concern us here. We will attempt to derive maximum life force from the air through the aid of our breathing exercises, and from food by adopting the Yogic principles of nutrition. We will also make certain suggestions regarding sleep, water, and sun. However, as I implied above, once having derived the necessary life force from these sources, we must make certain that we retain it in sufficient amounts and that it is allowed to circulate freely and fully throughout the organism. In other words, the flow of the life force must not be inhibited; we can undertake certain Yoga techniques to help insure this free flow.

Tension, tightness, and stiffness are major inhibitors of the circulation of life force. In Yoga we believe that wherever you find yourself stiff or tight, you will also experience *tension;* it is at these tension points, regardless of where they are, that the life force is blocked, that energy is trapped. For our purposes in this study let us consider tension, tightness, stiffness as one condition. Our remedy for this condition: *methodical stretching.* Stretching is so effective in removing tension that is continually accumulating that I suggest that you do it throughout the day!

At this point we will perform two such methodical stretching exercises. Let me place these stretching movements in perspective with regard to our morning routine. You have slept for approximately eight hours. Your breathing has been shallow (which is natural), your circulation has slowed (which is natural), and your body has become stiff (which is also natural). The quickest way to "wake up" is to counteract these conditions. We have already done our deep, complete breathing, and now we will gently accelerate the circulation and simultaneously eliminate the stiffness, tightness, knots, and cramps with a few minutes of stretching.

Are you aware that almost all **Yoga** movements are extremely gentle and executed in slow motion? There is absolutely no jumping or leaping about, no huffing and puffing, no exertion or strain, no perspiration and exhaustion. Such things are totally irrelevant and unnecessary to accomplish our Yogic objectives. If it is your custom to engage in other forms of morning exercises, in weight lifting, calisthenics, and the like, you can certainly feel free to continue them; Yoga will not be an impediment to any of these; on the contrary, it will improve all physical activities, including your golf, bowling, and tennis game, your ballet or judo studies. But if you want to be able to evaluate the full value of Yoga, you should temporarily discontinue other forms of exercising including jogging and the various systems of calisthenics. Swimming, bicycling, ballet, and walking for exercise may be continued.

Also, if you suffer from arthritis, bursitis, or other conditions of the joints, you may very well find that the Yoga movements are the most effective natural things you have ever done. I say this because so many class students and television viewers have reported to me that they experienced anything from minor to the most dramatic improvements in their conditions. It seems that the very slow, cautious *self-manipulation* of the joints have, within the course of patient practice, effected these improvements. Consult your physician first and obtain his approval. But arthritis or not, if you find your body becoming persistently stiff in a particular area, it may indicate trouble in the future and a definite deterrent to the free flow of the life force now. I state unequivocally that there has never been a more comprehensive system of body movements for eliminating tension and stiffness than those that comprise the study of *Hatha Yoga*.

LEG CLASP
(1 minute)

When you have completed your 5 rounds of CHARG-ING—COMPLETE BREATHING, you move directly into this exercise.

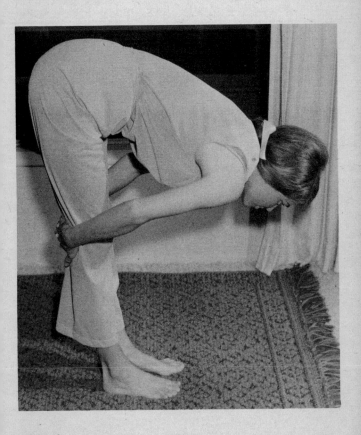

FIG. 6
Bend forward slowly and clasp your hands firmly just below your knees.

FIG. 7

Brace your clasped hands against the backs of your knees and very slowly and very cautiously bend your trunk to that point where you begin to feel a slight strain and stop. Do not attempt to go beyond this point. Do not strain. Simply stop all motion and hold your extreme position with your head down.

Hold for a count of 10. Allow the blood to flow into your head.

Relax your trunk and slowly return to the position of Fig. 6, but keep your hands clasped. Rest a moment.

Repeat and do 3 in all.

Unclasp your hands and very slowly straighten to the upright position. Rest for a few moments without fidgeting.

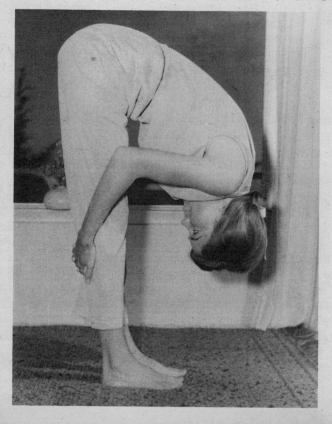

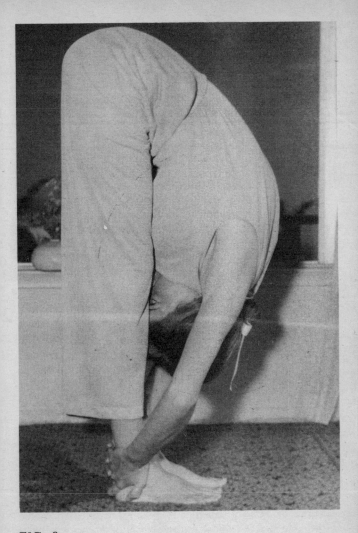

FIG. 8

The Yoga exercises are wonderfully *progressive*. Simply by following these directions, making certain not to strain or go beyond that point where the position is comfortable and by making sure to hold your extreme position exactly

21

for the indicated count with as little motion as possible, you will find each day allows you to extend your extreme position a little farther. Very soon you will achieve an advanced position that in the beginning you may have thought far beyond your capability.

This illustration depicts such an advanced position. Note that the hands are now clasped at the heels and the head touches the legs below the knees. The spine experiences no strain because each vertebra has, in turn, received sufficient stress through the patient holding of each day's extreme position. (Once gained it becomes relatively easy to retain this flexibility for your entire life.)

A flexible, elastic spine is the "key" to the free flow of the life force. According to Yogic theory, it is also the key to remaining youthful in body and mind. If you've seen my television programs, you know how often I try to impress this upon my viewers by repeating the axiom, "You're as young as your spine is flexible." Young people who have allowed their spines to grow inflexible come to my classes; they move in a certain stiff, adhesive manner and consequently have acquired an aura of premature aging. You can actually see their youthfulness return week by week as they exchange stiffness for flexibility and become limber through their Yoga practice. In another book I have explained in detail the seven major characteristics of youth and how it is possible to regain them regardless of age.* It is not unusual for grandparents who practice Yoga to show far more flexibility than their grandchildren!

RISHI'S EXERCISE
(2 minutes)

Many years ago, during my travels in quest of Yogic knowledge, I met a most impressive Hindu who was part-time successful businessman and part-time Yoga instructor. Subsequently, I spent some months with him at his private

---

*Hittleman, *Be Young with Yoga* (New York: Paperback Library, 1971).

retreat in the Santa Ynez mountains of California, and it was he who first afforded me an insight into the practical possibilities of applying Yoga during business hours. Among various techniques that he utilized in this manner was the Headstand. His activities necessitated extensive travel by auto, and while the distances were usually very long he would drive them by himself, nonstop. In addition to the breathing exercises that he did for revitalizing while driving, every few hundred miles he would stop in an isolated area, walk away from the highway, and perform a five minute Headstand. He maintained that this proved so refreshing he could easily drive the next few hundred miles without fatigue. I can tell you from my own experience that this is absolutely true; the Headstand is every bit as effective for driving endurance as he stated and as effective in refreshing the brain as Yogis have always claimed. (I might suggest that if you ever want to test this theory with regard to your own driving, make sure you get well away from the road as the highway patrolmen seem to take a dim view of the driver of a parked vehicle being discovered in an inverted posture.)

When this gentleman was a young man not yet practicing Yoga, he discovered that one side of his body was more developed than the other and the corresponding leg was longer. This imbalance, which appeared to be structural, was a source of great disturbance. Eventually, a friend of his family advised him to see a particular *Hatha* Yogi who had an excellent reputation for physical therapy. From this Yogi he learned a posture that he claimed was instrumental in remedying the condition: it is an ingenious stretching movement that acts to balance or equalize the sides and shape the trunk and limbs in a most desirable manner. We will now perform this posture; because the gentleman from whom I learned it was called "Rishi" (great teacher) by his students, I have named this series of movements "Rishi's Exercise."

Remain facing east. You have completed the Leg Clasp and rested a few moments without fidgeting and without allowing your mind to wander. If you find you're involved with other thoughts, bring the mind back gently but firmly to the business at hand.

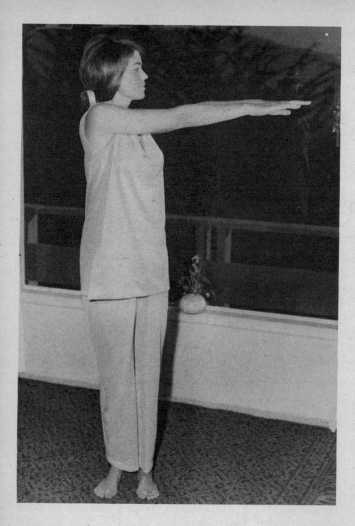

FIG. 9

In a standing position, with your heels together, slowly raise your arms so that the hands meet in front of you at eye level. Fix your gaze on the backs of your hands and very slowly turn left to the ninety degree position.

FIG. 10

Study the illustration carefully. Your right hand moves very slowly down your right leg and holds your right upper calf firmly. Your left arm moves behind you and your gaze must follow your left hand.

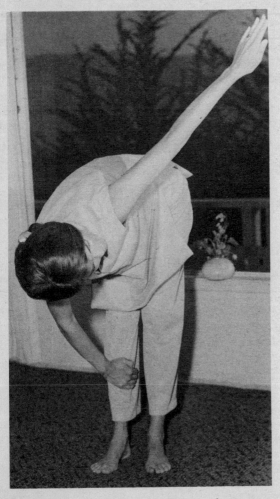

FIG. 11

Your left arm moves to the overhead position (or as far as you can bring it without strain), and your gaze remains fixed on the back of your left hand. Hold without motion for a count of 10.

Now slowly raise your trunk and bring your arms back into the position where your hands meet in front of you at eye level.

Slowly twist to the *right* and perform the identical movements to the right side. Hold for 10.

Slowly straighten to the upright position and repeat on the *left* side. Perform 3 times on both sides.

Lower your arms to the sides and relax briefly, without fidgeting.

FIG. 12

With a little practice you should be able to attain this extreme position with your hand down to your heel area. But remember our "progressive" concept: there is no rush to accomplish any extreme position, and there is never to be any strain experienced in attempting the more advanced positions.

Let me remind you that we want to keep our minds free from the mundane thoughts of our daily activities throughout this brief ten minute routine. We must not permit ourselves to perform the movements of these exercises in a semiautomatic fashion, that is, where the body moves but the mind wanders elsewhere. There are systems of exercising that are so inane and boring, the movements so uncomfortable, that the instructor will actually make the attempt to distract your mind through talking, music, and the like. The exact opposite is the case in Yoga. Here we put aside all other thoughts so that we may concentrate as fully and deeply as possible on the movements we are performing. We actually attempt to merge with the movements; we feel, sink into, and become the movements. It is as though we are utterly immersed in a series of beautiful, slow-motion dances, and, indeed, I would suggest that you think of yourself as a dancer here and move with as much grace, poise, and balance as you can muster.

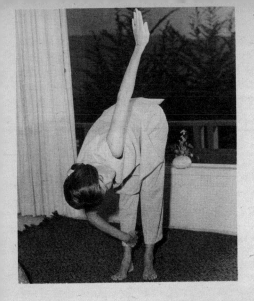

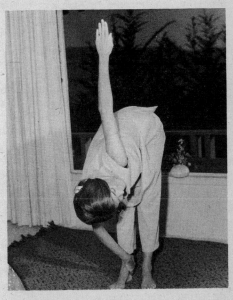

Think gracefully, move gracefully with loose sweeping motions. Don't be afraid to exaggerate such motions. Nobody is watching you and you'll be surprised at how this type of movement can improve your appearance and co-ordination in your general activities, extending even to the way in which you walk, do your housework, or play golf. Concentrate on your movements.

ABDOMINAL LIFTS
(3 minutes)

If I told you to "exercise your liver, spleen, stomach, kidneys, heart, thyroid, and brain," would you know what to do? We usually don't think about methodically exercising or stimulating various organs and glands through our own movements because we've never been told that it's possible to do so. Yet it certainly makes sense that if we are going to become involved in a program of physical fitness, it should be a truly comprehensive one, including consideration of the organs and glands—consideration that is almost totally lacking in the various systems of calisthenics and "body building."

So we come now to that fascinating, invaluable aspect of *Hatha* Yoga that I designate as "internal exercising." We will do many internal exercises in the course of our day's Yoga routines that directly affect the organs and glands. The most obvious and immediately effective of these is the Abdominal Lift. With this lifting movement we will reach the stomach, colon, intestines, liver, kidneys, gall bladder, and pancreas! This exercise is very valuable for the sedentary worker: these movements will enable him to give conscious attention to those organs and glands that are almost never stimulated in the course of his usual day's activities.

We perform the Abdominal Lifts soon after arising because they are hygienic in nature and among other benefits stimulate, through natural movements, the organs of elimination. Along these lines I would make a suggestion that has proven very helpful to many of my students: if you

28

have a problem in proper elimination drink six ounces of cool water immediately upon getting out of bed. The water will be well into your stomach by the time you are ready to do the Abdominal Lifts. These movements, together with the water, will aid in cleansing and elimination.

Other major benefits that result from this exercise are the loss of inches in the abdominal area and the maintenance of resilience of the abdominal wall, helping to prevent a prolapse (dropping) of the abdomen.

Having completed Rishi's Exercise and rested a few moments without fidgeting, we go on to the Abdominal Lift. First, we must again practice to gain some definite control of the abdominal muscles so that we can contract and distend the abdomen even more acutely than we did in our Breathing Routine. The movements of Figs. 13, 14, and 15 can be done in a seated position until mastered.

FIG. 13

Sit in a simple cross-legged posture and rest your hands on your knees. Fix your attention fully on your abdominal muscles. Now contract these muscles as much as possible and try to create a fairly deep "hollow" in your abdominal area. Hold whatever contraction you attain (even one inch) for a count of three. You can breathe normally during this hold.

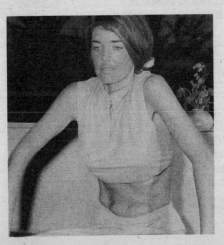

FIG. 14

Now use the same set of muscles to forcefully and quickly push the abdomen out as far as possible. This is not simply a relaxing of the abdomen; it is a forceful, sudden pushing or "snapping" out of the abdomen.

Without pause repeat these contracting, distending movements at least ten times or until you tire. Rest a few moments and repeat the series. During the first few days you should devote about two minutes of practice to this. Even the slightest contraction and distension will begin to strengthen these muscles and enable you to make real progress within a few days. Remember that you will lose inches and gain firmness with this exercise, but the most important thing is to gain the necessary control so that the following movement can be executed properly.

FIG. 15

Study the illustration. This is the objective of our previous practice. Note that now the abdomen is not merely contracted but is raised, lifted. This raise requires two things: control of the muscles and the emptying of the lungs through a deep and complete *exhalation* before the lift is attempted. You cannot raise the abdomen into this position unless the lungs are empty and remain empty for the duration of the lift.

Therefore, you must now exhale deeply and keep the air out of your lungs. This creates the necessary vacuum. Now imagine that you're going to take a deep breath from the pit of your stomach; use your abdominal muscles as you would your lungs, so that the abdomen is "sucked" inward and upward (of course, no air is permitted to enter; this is a deep "breath" with the abdominal muscles, not with the lungs).

Hold the lift for a second or two and then quickly and forcefully "snap" your abdomen outward as we practiced previously.

Repeat 10 times without pause; then inhale deeply and relax about 5 seconds. Do not let your mind wander.

Now perform the next deep *exhalation* and repeat the movements.

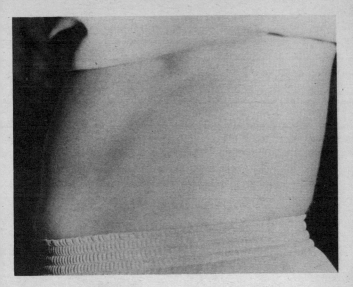

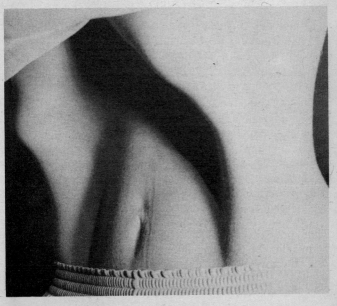

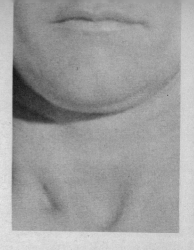

FIG. 16

A good indication that you have achieved the ultimate lift is this indentation that will occur in the jugular notch (at the base of your throat). You can test your progress by occasionally feeling this area with your fingers.

It is probable that I have instructed several million people in this exercise through my classes, television programs, and newspaper articles. I know there is great variety in the way students have caught on to the technique of the lift. Some learn it instantaneously, others require some weeks or longer. With sufficient practice the moment arrives when you simply get the "knack" of the lift, as you might get the knack of maintaining your balance on a bicycle. Actually, in this exercise your practice to do the movements properly is as important as the final accomplishment. You will be continually benefiting from each practice session with this exercise regardless of the depth of your contraction or lift. So don't be discouraged if, as with our breathing routine, success is not immediate. You will attain the position in time and once you do you can never lose it; this is a technique with lifetime benefits.

Once the lift is perfected or, at least, you have made good progress with your contractions, it should be performed in the Standing and All Fours positions that follow. Each of these places different organs and glands in positions where they can be stimulated. The sitting position that we use for learning is no longer necessary.

FIG. 17

Study the illustration. In a standing position with your feet apart, imagine that you are going to squat onto your heels, but only go a few inches down and stop . Knees are bent slightly outward, hands are pressed firmly against upper thighs, fingers (including thumbs) are together and turned inward. (The correct positions of all of these exercises are of paramount importance, so do them correctly, with style, and don't ever become lackadaisical. The practice of Yoga is that of an art form.)

Assume this position, exhale deeply, and perform your 10 lifts (or deep contractions).

Following the 10th, straighten to the upright position, inhale deeply, and relax a few moments without fidgeting.

Repeat and do 3 rounds in all (30 lifts).

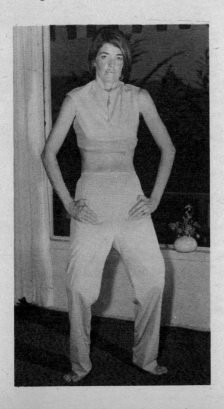

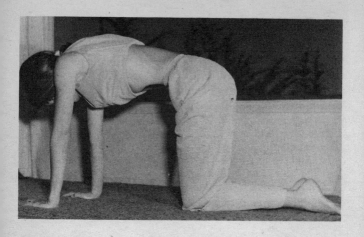

FIG. 18

Assume the All Fours position with your knees together, fingers and hands placed exactly as illustrated, and head down.

Exhale deeply and perform 10 lifts.

Following the 10th, remain as you are but inhale deeply and relax a few moments without fidgeting.

Repeat and do 3 rounds in all (30 lifts).

Summary:

Standing position—30 lifts (3 groups of 10)

Sitting position— 30 lifts (3 groups of 10)

Remember that the movements do not constitute a continual rolling of the abdomen; there must be the slightest pause between each lift and each "snap" out. Practice to make your movements rhythmic, sharp, definitive. Concentrate fully on what you're doing.

LOTUS

The two postures that are immediately associated with Yoga and are surprisingly familiar to those who are otherwise totally ignorant of what is involved in this ancient science are the Headstand and the Lotus. To the uninitiated these postures appear, of course, peculiar, curious, exotic, bizarre. At the root of the incredulity expressed by the uninformed is the apparent *discomfort* of these positions. "Why in the world should anyone want to invert his body and purposely allow the blood to run into his head?" Or, "Why should I subject my poor legs to those strenuous contortions necessary for the Lotus posture?" These questions are always put to me with a sad shake of the head and implicit is the train of thought, "These poses represent the ultimate in discomfort; intentionally subjecting oneself to discomfort suggests illness or insanity; Yogis, therefore, are probably nuts." It is with this type of reasoning that untold millions of Westerners formerly dismissed Yoga as a bizarre cult, an inexplicable passing fad. But Yoga is not a fad, nor will it pass in the foreseeable future. On the contrary, interest has increased to an extraordinary degree and will, I am certain, continue to grow. In this age of re-examination of the ancient sciences, people (and especially young people) have begun to ask, "Why?" *"Why* do Yogis stand on their heads?" *"Why* do Yogis sit in that strange cross-legged position?" The reasons are as fascinating as anything one could hope to learn regarding the human organism.

The Headstand will be discussed and learned later. But let us determine here why the Lotus position has been utilized for at least as long as man has recorded history. This last exercise of our brief "Arising" routine can actually be thought of as a "mental" exercise. I have stated that the breathing and stretching movements we just completed will serve to awaken and raise the vibrations of your body, insure the free flow of the life force, and enable you to become more "in touch" with yourself. These same physical movements will also help to put you in good spirits emotionally and make your mind alert (especially if you concentrate fully on the movements as suggested). This is true because in the study of Yoga we know that there is no separation of body and mind. The organism is one entity; whatever affects your body must have a corresponding effect on your mind and vice versa.

With the exercises just performed, we have concentrated primarily on the physical aspect of the organism. Now we want to spend a few minutes in raising our mental vibrations, in "tuning in" to our higher consciousness, to the spiritual aspect of our existence. We would then hope to sustain this sense of elevation throughout the day. There are a number of classical techniques that Yogis use to accomplish this. Most of them are very old and have been perfected through the centuries so that we can predict, with a fair degree of accuracy, that they will accomplish what they have been designed for. Which of these are used is dependent upon one's temperament, natural inclinations, stage of spiritual development, and other factors that are taken into consideration by one's Guru. Similar to the physical exercies, these techniques begin simply and gradually become increasingly complex in an extremely progressive fashion, as more refined levels of consciousness are attained. The practice of these exercises is referred to under the general heading of "meditation"; in the serious study of Yoga, as well as in all systems of metaphysics, meditation is indispensable.

To derive the greatest benefits from meditation, however brief or lengthy the session may be, your mind must be absolutely free so that it may be devoted exclusively to the meditation exercise. In other words, we must attempt to reduce the possibilities of distractions to a minimum. If you are able to select a quiet, private place for meditation, the external disturbances are minimized. But of equal importance are the internal disturbances, most of which are fairly subtle: whenever the body moves the mind is disturbed because the two are inseparable; if the body is uncomfortable the mind is forced to acknowledge this discomfort; if the senses are preoccupied (if, for example, something catches your eye or ear) the mind is preoccupied since the mind and the senses are one; how you breathe directly relates to how you think, so if your breathing is erratic, quick, or otherwise irregular the mind follows suit. The ancient Gurus were acutely aware of these problems and, through painstaking experiments that were probably carried out over many centuries, arrived at a solution that has never been improved upon—the Lotus posture.

The Lotus, when perfected, enables you to sit for extended periods of time almost completely motionless because of the stability of the posture. The legs are placed in a position where they are literally "locked" out of the way; the trunk and head are balanced and well supported; therefore, the mind is not distracted through movement or discomfort. Further, simply sitting correctly in this posture has a remarkable, almost magical quieting effect on the senses and produces an automatic slowing of the breathing process. Although at this point in our program we are speaking of only a two minute interval of meditation, there may come a time soon when you will want to increase this period and then the full value of the Lotus will be realized.

I have had too much experience with teaching the Lotus to tell you that you're going to have an easy time with it, but my experience also enables me to state that within a few weeks of beginning your Lotus practice, you should accomplish a satisfactory position. Indeed, depending upon the structure and flexibility of your legs, you might do a very respectable Half or even Full Lotus on your very first try. But the degree of attainment is absolutely unimportant in the beginning stages; the essential thing is the patient practice that will lead to success. Remember that there are many benefits for the knees, ankles, and feet inherent in this practice.

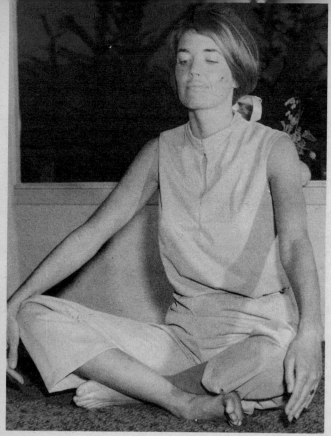

FIG. 19

Sit facing east. This is the cross-legged posture. People who are overweight, elderly, or exceptionally stiff may have to begin with this position to help limber their legs, knees, and ankles. Your ankles are crossed and your legs are drawn in as far as possible. Keep your trunk erect but relaxed. Your knees, which may be raised some distance from the floor in the beginning, will gradually lower. You can have your right leg on top one day and reverse the position on the next, placing the left leg on top. Lower your eyes but don't close them. Rest your wrists on your knees.

FIG. 20

Preparation for the Half-Lotus. Your left heel is placed as close to the body as possible.

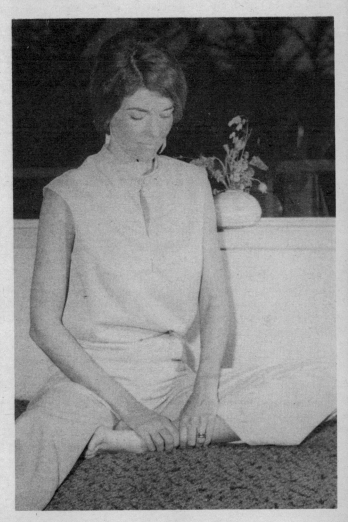

FIG. 21

The right foot is placed either on the left thigh or in the cleft of the left leg, whichever is more comfortable. The trunk remains erect but relaxed; eyes are lowered (not closed) and the wrists rest on the knees.

Try the Half-Lotus with the legs reversed on alternate days to develop flexibility in both legs.

Don't be concerned if the knee of the leg on top is raised a fair distance from the floor. You will be surprised at how quickly it begins to lower of its own accord. Make no attempt to push or force this knee down. It won't stay.

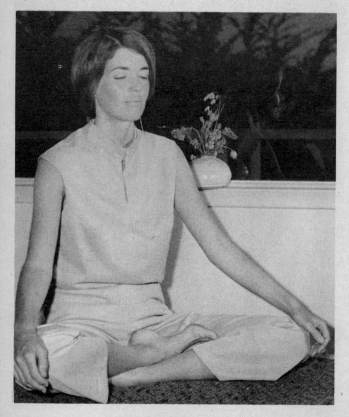

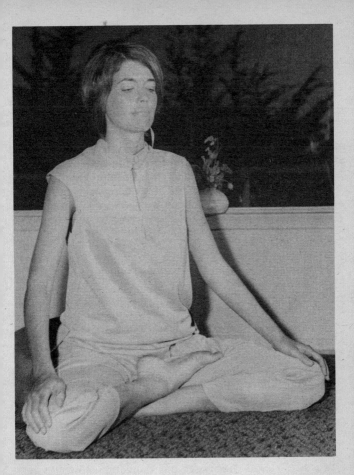

FIG. 22

If you find your knees very high in the Half-Lotus, you might try sitting on the edge of one or two pillows. This will automatically bring your knees closer to the floor. (Instructions for the Full Lotus will come during our "Weekend" routine.)

So you are now seated in either the simple cross-legged or Half-Lotus posture. We are going to perform 2 minutes of meditation.

MANTRA MEDITATION
(2 minutes)

There is a branch of Yoga that deals with sound vibrations, particularly those produced by the voice. Certain single sounds and groups of sounds, when uttered in a specific way, infuse us with a unique type of etheric energy and act to raise our vibrations. These sounds are known as *mantras*. In India the Guru determines which mantras are to be used by the student to help him achieve a particular objective. For our purposes here we can take advantage of that which is acknowledged by all gurus to be the most powerful of the *mantras*—a two letter word "OM" that is pronounced "Oooooo-Mmmmmm." (The "O" is as in "oh.") This is the universal *mantra;* it has no religious connotations and is chanted by students of Yoga through the world who have many different religious affiliations. It is this dynamic, energizing *mantra* that we will now employ for our brief morning meditation exercise.

You are seated in either the simple cross-legged or Half-Lotus posture. Remember that your spine is straight but your trunk relaxed, your nose is in a straight line with your navel, your hands rest easily on your knees, and your eyelids are lowered, not completely closed (you are looking into your upper lids). This position of the eyes is maintained during meditation so that you do not associate the practice with sleep (eyes closed), nor will your mind be distracted by the eyes alighting on various objects (eyes open).

Slowly inhale a Complete Breath as we have learned previously but do not raise your shoulders. Now, in a low, steady, controlled voice use half the air in your lungs to produce the sound "O" (with the lips shaped in the form of an "o") and the remaining half to slowly produce the sound "M." The vibrations of the "M" sound with the lips pressed lightly together should be strong enough to be felt throughout the head and chest. Your attention is fully focused on these sounds; they must not be produced automatically while your mind is allowed to wander elsewhere. The "OM" mantra is chanted with feeling and intensity;

it has the quality of an oratorio. When you run out of breath, take another Complete Breath and repeat. If each repetition does not last at least 10 seconds, you're going too fast.

Perform 7 times slowly in a low, steady, controlled voice. Seven repetitions should require approximately 1 minute, 45 seconds. Spend the next 15 to 30 seconds sitting very quietly, breathing normally, and becoming aware of the tremendously uplifting effect this *mantra* has had upon your organism.

This completes the "Arising" routine.

TWO YOGA HYGIENIC TECHNIQUES

Now that you have completed the routine your next activity will probably be to wash. The Yogi, as you might imagine, is extremely fastidious about his hygiene and there are several points of a hygienic nature that we shall consider here.

In addition to brushing the teeth, the Yogi believes it is also important to clean the tongue, that is, to remove the excess coating that accumulates during sleep. If you think for a moment you will probably agree that this is a sensible and healthful practice. Here is the method: obtain any metal instrument with which you can gently scrape the tongue without any possibility of injury. The edge of a spoon or a dull butter knife is often put aside for this purpose. Go over the tongue several times scraping it gently from the root to the tip. Your mouth and breath will feel much the better for this practice.

The Yogi also cleans the nasal passages each morning with a solution of salt water. Not only is congestion relieved, but the nasal passages are more fully opened, and I definitely believe that there is a positive effect produced on the mucous membranes. A Mexican Yogi whom I met in Guadalajara told me that he had not caught cold in 30 years and that he attributed this primarily to his daily inhalation of salt water. Here is the procedure: to a glass of warm water add two teaspoons of table salt.* Stir. Hold the glass in your right hand and pour a small amount of the solution into your left hand. Put the glass down. Bring the left hand up to your left nostril and simultaneously close the right nostril with your right index finger *(Fig. 23)*. Very gently sniff the solution into the left nostril; about 3 to 4 gentle inhalations will consume the water in your hand. Do not expel. Almost all of the water should remain in the nostril. Now follow the same procedure for the right nostril. At this point close both nostrils, lower your head (as illustrated in *Fig. 24*), and hold for approximately 15 seconds, which you can count. This allows the solution to pass into the sinuses. Now raise your head, press the right nostril closed, and *gently* expel the water from the left nostril. Two to three gentle but firm blows will clear the nostril *(Fig. 25)*. Do the same with the right nostril. Then repeat the entire procedure once again. I find this practice highly beneficial in cold or damp climates particularly during winter months.

As I have indicated, Yogis go to great lengths to insure cleanliness of every part of their bodies. In India today ingenious techniques that were developed by Yogis in very ancient times for the washing of each orifice, the cleansing of the respiratory tract, stomach, and intestines are still used. Because of our immediate access to bathing facilities, particularly the bath and shower, and because our food and drinking water are relatively free from harmful bacteria, these additional and elaborate cleansing procedures need not concern us here.

---

*If the solution proves too strong for you simply decrease the amount of salt.

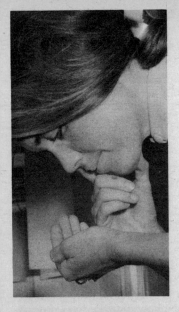

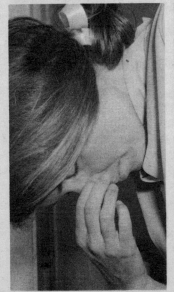

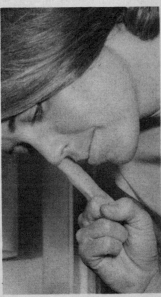

BREAKFAST

(See the following section on "Nutrition")

NUTRITION

I have been lecturing on the subject of Yoga Nutrition for twenty years and in preparing this chapter I have gone through my various notes for these lectures, back to the very first one. I find that the most significant changes I have made in my lectures through the years are of a negative nature, that is, I have had to include more and more foods *not to eat,* methods of cooking *not to use,* advertising promises *not to believe.* I now list almost twice as many foods on my "don't" chart as I did twenty years ago. This is because as the grower, producer, packager, and manufacturer have learned how to make food processing more profitable for their companies, the food with which they are tampering not only continues to lose more and more of its nutritional value but possibly becomes harmful.

Twenty years ago I met with great incredulity when I would explain that many foods that were mainstays of the national diet were, due to processing and additives, low in nutritional value and might even be responsible for much of the ill health that prevailed throughout the nation. Most people simply could not believe this. Their general response was: if there was anything wrong with the way food was grown, harvested, shipped, packaged, and stored, the government would intervene. In those years also I never gave a lecture without cautioning people against smoking and telling them of the numerous dangers that were inherent in cigarettes. I remember one outraged man questioning me from the audience. "If smoking was harmful," he said, "do you think Uncle Sam would let us do it?" He reinforced his argument by citing the number of physicians who smoked, including his own doctor. Yes, ironically Uncle Sam and the doctors *have* finally told the nation to quit smoking—about seventy years late and only when the deaths from lung cancer and other respiratory and heart diseases grew at such an alarming rate that they were impossible to ignore any longer. I have no doubt that the time must come when the government will be forced to ban dozens of chemicals that now adulterate our food and will seriously investigate the denaturing of food by the various processes to which it is currently subjected. But we cannot predict the cost in health and lives that may be involved before this comes about. However, the change in response even to my own lectures during the past few years is highly encouraging because now people are really listening. The efforts of hundreds of nutritionists and crusaders for "truth in selling" have begun to effect some major re-evaluations on the part of the consumer. He is at least learning to read the labels to determine what additives (chemicals) are in the products; he is questioning the wisdom of "refining" and other processes that remove the vital nutrients from the food; many consumers, unable or unwilling to continue to pay the outrageous prices for their cannibalism, are eating a lot less or no meat and finding it very healthful in many respects; millions of young people, impervious to the slogans of Madison Avenue, refuse to eat denatured products and grow and sell their own organic food. Many positive signs that are too numerous to cite here are, for the population in general, encouraging. As the consumer becomes well informed, we will certainly see him outraged; this will put heavy pressure on both the producer and the government, and the necessary vital reforms will be instituted.

We must now, however, leave generalities (in speaking about the "population-at-large") and get down to specifics that concern you as a Yoga student. Correct diet constitutes an indispensable aspect of Yoga, so while this is not a book on nutrition, it is, nonetheless, necessary to present the reader with an outline, in the form of lists and menus, to indicate the type of foods that comprise the various meals of the Yogi's diet. In this book I do not explain in detail the reasons for including or excluding foods. The reader, if interested, will find such explanations in those of my books that are devoted to nutrition. But you do not necessarily need to be fully informed about these technicalities to experiment with and benefit from the Yoga nutrition suggestions in the following pages.

Above I stated that the major changes in my lectures over a period of two decades were primarily of a negative nature, that is, more and more of *what not to do.* You may think, "With the incredible body of knowledge that is added to any study over a period of ten years, how is it that in twenty years significant developments have not occurred in Yoga nutrition?" Well, minor things have evolved, but the one guiding principle remains the same; it has been so for an untold number of centuries and will never change; its timeless quality is what commands and justifies our trust. This guiding principle consists of the following question: "How much life force (prana) is in this food I am about to eat?" Everything in the science of Yoga nutrition evolves from this question, which, in turn, implies these questions: "Is this food pure, unadulterated, free from additives? To what extent has it been tampered with, refined, processed? How shall I best prepare it so that it retains its life force?" Because the Yogi's key to all decisions regarding the selection and preparation of food revolves around life force, the diet of today is essentially not much different than that prescribed by the Gurus many centuries ago.

All foods contain some life force; those that contain the most of this element are of the greatest value to us. In the following pages you will find lists of foods for breakfast, lunch, dinner, and snacks. The foods listed are those that, from our Yogic viewpoint, are highest in life force. Because of the life-force concept you will find many foods that have been important to you (or rather, important to your taste buds or to the artificial stimulation of your nervous system) not included. Meats are excluded because their life force is minimal: they come from slaughtered creatures, the quality of their protein is, from our viewpoint, low, and their nutritional properties highly questionable. (This is aside from any philosophical or spiritual considerations.) No refined sugar or flour products are included; refining removes the "germ," the essential life force of the grain. The detrimental properties of refined sugar and refined flour products (breads, cakes, candies, colas, to name just a few) are becoming better known all the time. Coffee and alcohol, which artifically stimulate the nervous system and are absolutely additive—as much as any "hard" drug, withdrawal symptoms included—are in direct opposition to the controlled, naturally calm state of the organism that is one of our Yogic objectives. We attempt to include a minimum of foods in this diet that contain the various chemicals additives for reasons that are shocking, but that require more pages than this book permits. I have detailed these reasons in other writings.*

We prefer dairy products in which the butter fat content is as low as possible, a minimum of strong seasonings and condiments in all foods (the usual table salt is supplanted with vegetable salt), and almost no canned products since we believe that life force is seriously reduced in a food that has been sealed in a can and often remains there for months or even years. With regard to cooking methods we suggest light steaming and broiling in place of boiling and frying and stainless steel cookware rather than aluminum and "teflon."

You may use as many or as few of these suggestions and Yoga menus as you wish. As with the exercises you will benefit from whatever Yoga nutrition principles you do apply. Hopefully, you might undertake the entire program for several weeks so that you would be able to evaluate fully the effect that these more natural, more organic, higher life-force foods have upon you. But to judge the entire program fairly you must adopt it completely for a minimum of three weeks. During these three weeks you will begin to experience the light, clear, alert, invigorated state that a diet of exclusively high life-force foods produces. If this state becomes meaningful to you, you will be induced to continue with the Yoga diet (in many different forms and variations) for some time to come. This would be the ideal situation. However, if you cannot dedicate yourself fully to the program at this time,

*Hittleman, *Yoga Natural Foods Cookbook* (New York: Bantam Books, 1970).

use it partially, one or two meals a day, according to the menus offered. Let me emphasize that these menus are meant to serve only as samples; the food lists for the various meals will provide the sources for an infinite variety of menus.

You should always remember that what you eat determines to a great extent how you feel and how you function. The Yogi is acutely aware of this fact and to him nutrition is very serious business. To derive the most amount of *prana* from what is eaten with the least expenditure of digestive energy, to feel light and healthy in body, to be alert and optimistic—these are all possible with the aid of Yoga nutrition. Several hundred thousands of my students know that this is so. Whatever extra efforts you may have to make to obtain high life-force foods and prepare them correctly, or to seek out these more natural foods when eating out, will be well rewarded.

LISTS OF FOODS AND SAMPLE MENUS

Foods are listed under the headings of those meals at which you are likely to use them most or where we suggest they be used. However, this is simply a convenient manner of listing; any food may be used at any meal, according to your desires.

Foods to Be Consumed Extremely Sparingly or Eliminated Entirely from All Meals

The usual high-fat, homogenized, pasteurized milks
Buttermilk
Sour cream
Cream cheese
All highly salted and spiced cheeses
All yogurts flavored with fruits and syrups

Butter

Coffee

Tea (the usual commercial brands)

Alcoholic beverages (if you must, use very sparingly; wines are best)

Colas and all syrup drinks (including the "substitute sugar" colas)

Ice cream and ice cream beverages

All bottled, frozen, and canned fruits and fruit juices with "sugar added" or "in heavy syrup"

Salt and, as much as possible or practical, all salted products

All "smoked" products

All hot spices and condiments (such as chili peppers; sauces such as Tabasco, Worcestershire)

All refined flour products (such as white bread, dry cereals, most cakes, cookies, pastas)

Meat, poultry, fish (as an experiment for, let us say, a three week trial period as explained previously in this section)

White rice

All fried, overcooked, greasy foods

All refined sugar and refined sugar products (cakes, cookies, pies, puddings, candies, jellies, jams)

All syrups

All chemical sugar substitutes

All "instant breakfasts"; wafers, powders, tablets, referred to as "low-calorie" and/or "high-protein" products

As many canned products as possible (the amount of life force that remains in a vacuum sealed can is highly questionable)

Foods for Breakfast

All fresh fruit juices (use the frozen ones sparingly)

All fresh fruits in season (use the frozen ones sparingly)

All *whole grain* (unrefined) hot or cold cereals, including brown rice

All *whole grain* (unrefined, unbleached flour) breads,
crackers, muffins

Margarine (polyunsaturated)

Milk (low-fat or nonfat)

Eggs (sparingly; preferably boiled only)

Herb teas (dozens of delicious and healthful ones are
available at health food stores)

Low or noncaffein beverages

For sweetening at all meals:

Molasses

Honey (uncooked, unbleached)

Raw sugar

Carob powder (at health food stores)

Brown sugar (only slightly superior to white, refined
sugar)

Sample Breakfast Menus

(1)

Fresh orange juice (that
you squeeze yourself)

Steamed brown rice with
rasins, honey, nonfat milk

(3)

Baked apple (with honey
and yogurt topping if de-
sired)

2 boiled eggs

Whole grain toast with
margarine

(2)

Large serving of mixed
fresh fruit in season (peaches, apricots, strawberries;
topped with yogurt and
honey if desired)

Whole grain muffins with
margarine (or cashew but-
ter if preferred)

(4)

Grapefruit and orange sec-
tions

Whole grain hot cereal
with dates, nonfat milk, and
a natural sweetener

Fresh grape juice (made in
your blender using grapes
and a small amount of
spring water) or bottled,
unsweetened

Cold (dry) cereal made
from whole grains and
fruits (some brand names:
"Familia," "Swissy"—both
made in Switzerland and
available in many markets)
with nonfat milk and a
natural sweetener

All breakfasts can include a hot beverage at the conclusion
of the meal: herb tea or a low or noncaffein product.

Foods for "Snacks" (both A.M. and P.M.)

All fresh fruits in season (bananas, apples, pears, peaches,
cherries, grapes, plums, etc.)
All fresh fruit juices or unsweetened, bottled grape or
apple juice (take them to work in a thermos)
Nuts (preferably raw and unsalted, available in health
food stores): cashews, almonds, pecans, brazils,
walnuts, etc.
Seeds (preferably unroasted and unsalted): sunflower,
pumpkin, etc.
Yogurt (plain only; no flavors, no syrups)
All dried fruits that do not contain "sulphur dioxide used
as a preservative": dates, raisins, prunes, apricots,
peaches, currants
Whole grain crackers or cookies
Herb teas or noncaffein beverages (take them to work in
a thermos)

Foods for Lunch

All fresh vegetable juices (that you make yourself in your own vegetable juicer; take them in a thermos if necessary; a vegetable juicer is a valuable appliance and a good investment in health)

Fresh vegetable soups and broths (made from vegetables that are steamed, not boiled)

Salads (made from any combination of raw vegetables or fresh fruits or certain mixtures from both categories; see "Dinner" for complete listing of fruits and vegetables)

Oils for vegetable salad dressings and general cooking: safflower, sesame seed, pure olive (all polyunsaturated)

Condiments and seasonings: all edible herbs, vegetable salt (available at health food stores and some markets)

Cheeses: cottage (uncreamed or very lightly creamed), farmer, ricotta, Wisconsin cheddar (mild), jack, Swiss (mild)

Yogurt (plain only; no flavors, no syrups which destroy the entire value of yogurt)

Nut butters (sparingly): raw cashew, raw almond (available in health food stores)

Whole grain bread or crackers, with margarine if desired

Fresh fruit compote

Herb teas and low or noncaffein beverages

Sandwiches (on *whole grain* bread): cheese (as listed above); any combination of raw vegetables (lettuce, tomato, cucumbers, etc.); avocado; hard-boiled eggs; nut butter

Sample Lunch Menus

(1)

Fresh vegetable soup

Sandwich:* avocado, bean sprout, and tomato on whole grain bread

Yogurt (with honey and raisins if desired)

(2)

Fresh carrot and celery juice (from your own juicer)

Hard-boiled egg salad (with celery and homemade mayonnaise)

Whole grain bread or crackers with cheddar or Swiss cheese

Custard (made with nonfat milk and natural sweetening)

(3)

Apple juice (bottled, unsweetened, or from your own juicer)

Mushrooms and brown rice

Fresh fruit compote

(4)

Tomato stuffed with cottage or ricotta cheese and chives on romaine lettuce

Whole grain crackers or muffin

Stewed fruits: dried apricots, figs, and prunes soaked in water overnight. Top with yogurt

(5)

Salad: cheddar cheese, sliced figs, sliced apples, grapes, celery on a bed of lettuce (with homemade mayonnaise if desired)

Whole grain muffin with cashew butter

All lunches can include a hot beverage at the conclusion of the meal: herb tea or a low noncaffein product.

---

*Oatmeal, cracked-wheat, and soya flours make excellent sandwich breads.

Foods for Dinner

Fresh fruit or vegetable beverage

Fresh fruit or fresh fruit compote

Soups (made from any single vegetable or combination of vegetables listed below; also from the "legume" family: peas, lentils, many kinds of beans, including the soybean which is very rich in protein)

Salads (made from any combination of raw and/or lightly steamed vegetables listed below)

Entrées (using any of the foods listed previously and below: apples, apricots, artichokes, avocados, barley, beets, blueberries, broccoli, Brussels sprouts, cabbage, carrots, cauliflower, celery, cherries, cranberries, cucumbers, dandelion, eggplant, endive, garlic, grapefruit, grapes, green peas, green peppers, kale, leeks, lemons, lettuce, limes, melons, mustard greens, oranges, parsley, parsnips, peaches, pears, pineapples, plums, pomegranates, radishes, raspberries, rhubarb, rye, rutabagas, spinach, squash, strawberries, string beans, tangerines, tomatoes, turnips, watercress, all types of potatoes, all edible mushrooms, Swiss chard, all sprouts, onions

Note: the above listings include all members of a particular family, i.e., "cabbage" includes all types of cabbage—red, white, Chinese, etc.; "squash" includes zucchini, banana, etc.

Whole grain bread, crackers, muffins

Deserts: fresh fruit or fresh and dried fruit compote; pies, puddings, cakes, cookies (all very sparingly and using unrefined flour and the various natural elements previously listed such as natural sweeteners, brown rice, unsulphured dried fruits, nut butters, etc.)

Herb teas and low or noncaffein beverages

Sample Dinner Menus

(1)

Beet-yogurt blender drink made from beets, tomatoes, parsley, and yogurt

Casserole of steamed Chinese vegetables: Chinese cabbage, snow peas, bean sprouts, mustard greens

Baked yam with margarine

Grapes with mixed cheeses

(2)

Salad: stalks of raw celery, carrots, broccoli, green pepper, thin slices of cucumber and turnips; yogurt and chives or lemon and oil dressing

Whole wheat noodles with vegetarian tomato sauce and grated cheddar cheese

Watermelon sherbert (blend watermelon or other fresh or frozen fruit with sprig of mint; freeze)

(3)

Lentil soup

Baked eggplant with ricotta cheese and fresh tomato sauce (with onions and mushrooms)

Salad: shredded carrots, alfalfa sprouts, and chopped black olives on romaine lettuce; lemon and oil dressing

Orange gelatin with bananas (made with fresh squeezed orange juice and plain gelatin)

(4)

Fresh vegetable juice cocktail made in your juicer: ¼ cup parsley juice, ¼ cup carrot juice, ¼ cup celery juice, ¼ cup watercress ¼ cup spinach; mix or blend

Welsh rarebit made with natural cheddar cheese served over whole grain toast

Vegetable casserole: zucchini, tomatoes, onions

Baked apple slices, sprinkled with sesame seeds, cinnamon, honey, and lemon juice

Melon slices

Celery stalks stuffed with cottage cheese and chives

Soybean loaf

Steamed Swiss chard

Brown rice pudding

At all meals: whole grain bread, crackers, muffins
Beverages: cold—lemonade, limeade, orangeade, etc.
(freshly squeezed juices mixed with spring water and honey if desired)
hot—herb teas; low or noncaffein products

ON THE JOB

If your schedule follows that of most people, your next activity is the major one of your weekday: your work. Different types of work require, of course, different skills, different degrees of involvement, and different locations— home, office, field. However, from our Yogic viewpoint there are universal philosophical principles pertaining to work that deserve our attention because they often help one to gain a new and very meaningful perspective of his work.

You probably spend forty or more hours each week at your work, totaling another third of your life. (We mentioned before that sleep constituted the first third.) Yogis consider it essential that this large segment of one's lifetime that is spent in gaining the means to sustain life must also be productive in another equally important area: one's work, whatever it may be, must result in inner development and growth. Indeed, it is specifically stated in the Yoga texts that an essential aspect of self-realization can evolve only through the unique opportunity afforded by one's work!

Now it is a fact of life that the great majority of the Western world's population associates work with "original sin." Man has been cast out of the Garden and is forced to earn his bread in a tedious, generally unmeaningful way. Work, for most Americans and Europeans, represents the sacrifice of a certain portion of their lives so that the remaining portion may be sustained in a particular style. In other words, work is not an intrinsic part of the joy of living, a welcome opportunity for development, but a penance, a price to be paid so that another part of life may be salvaged. Therefore, if not consciously, then sub-consciously, most workers certainly identify as their "real life" that part that is lived during their leisure time, their nonworking hours rather than their jobs. This creates a continual schism, a split in which the worker feels his work not a part of, but apart from, his real life.

Our ultimate objective in the practice of Yoga is to achieve an integration, unity in our lives and spirit. Consequently, the aforementioned "split" is untenable. Our work *must* be agreeably incorporated into our lives; our working hours must be as productive to our inner lives as our leisure hours. But how shall this be accomplished? We have only to conjure up the image of ourselves at our work to recall instantaneously one or more of the following problems that it probably involves: the uninteresting nature of the work itself; the physical discomfort that is often experienced, especially by sedentary workers; the emotional disturbances that result from necessary relationships with other employees; the general frustrations from a position beneath our ability, lack of recognition, insufficient appreciation of our efforts, perhaps inadequate compensation, and others that you know all too well. In the face of such obstacles how is it possible that work can be conductive to growth?

I have stated previously that there are different types of Yoga designed for the various "paths" that one may find himself treading in the course of his evolution. In brief, *Hatha* Yoga is the physical system comprised of the exercises and the breathing techniques. *Raja* Yoga is concerned with the practice of quiet or inactive meditation. We have already practiced a little of both of these Yogas. Now we come to *Karma* Yoga, the Yoga that pertains to all of us who are involved in working, whatever the nature of the work may be. Certain guidelines were established by the ancient Gurus to help resolve the problems that they perceived were eternally inherent in work. These guidelines, set forth primarily in a beautifully poetic work that is the most widely read book in India—the *Bhagavad Gita*—are the essence of *Karma* Yoga, that method by which one's work serves as an avenue to self-realization. Let us examine the underlying principle of *Karma* Yoga.

The *Karma* Yogi learns through practice how in the performance of his duties he can eliminate the ego, the thought that "it is *I* who works." He learns how to become so completely immersed in his work that he *becomes* the work (as we become our movements during the physical exercises), and in this manner he allows the work to flow through him. He makes of himself an instrument that executes what needs to be done without the intervention of the ego, without the constant reminder *"I am; the worker."* This results in a wonderful sense of freedom, liberation from the tedium of the work concept. Outwardly all activities go on as before, but inwardly a transformation of the first order has occurred that permits the work to be performed with love in an egoless fashion. The moment the ego is removed from the picture many factors that have inhibited the efficiency of your work vanish. You remain perfectly aware of what you are doing; indeed, you are more aware and much more genuinely involved than was possible in the previous ego state; consequently, the work goes more smoothly and is accomplished with minimal mental or emotional strain.

How does one shake loose from the tentacles of the ego, of the constant reminder of "I"? Simply by desiring and practicing to do so! Before the start of each day's work, or as often as you can think about this during the day, dedicate your work to whatever you conceive of as the ultimate principle responsible for your existence: to Nature, to God, to Jesus, to Buddha. Implicit in this dedication is absolving yourself of not only whatever turmoil your labors entail, *but also the successful fruits of that labor*. Now this latter is a strange concept, isn't it? One can certainly understand the disavowal of whatever burns or pains may result from his efforts, but why would he want to remain unattached to the "fruits" of his labors? Isn't the enjoyment of one's achievements and successes what it's all about? Well, the fact is that the ego gains most of its strength and reality, and consequently is able to cause us the most pain and suffering, from our desires for success, from our need to achieve certain goals we have set for ourselves. We are driven by the fantasy that we will experience, taste, and luxuriate in our successes, but with some serious reflection it will be all too obvious that this need (which because of its illusory nature is seldom fulfilled and never satisfied) is largely responsible for many of our frustrations. We want the pleasure of success and accomplishment but not the pain of their opposites. Of course, this can never be, and it is of the greatest importance for us to know in the depth of our being that it can never be. We shall always have exactly as much failure and pain as we have success and pleasure. We shall suffer even in our moments of triumph because we know in our hearts that it's only a question of a short time until failure and pain reappear. The only permament solution, the only true security lies in simply allowing the structure of the "I," which we maintain with such great strain and at a woeful price, to collapse and disintegrate as completely as possible. And collapse it does (for its nature is illusory, without substance) the moment we are genuinely able to disassociate ourselves from it, to identify ourselves with our true nature, our real self.

"But," you may protest, "if I assume this nonattachment posture in my work, everything will suffer: I will lose interest, initiative, opportunity for advancement, and eventually probably the job itself." Not so! Whenever you gain the ability to "let go" of the ego (and please understand that this occurs intermittently, from time to time, during your initial experiments), you achieve a perspective, a certain balance, and most important of all, a love for and joy in your work that you have never possessed before. This is not the superficial, fleeting joy of material, temporal success. It is the pure joy that comes with no longer having to be concerned with the ego's concepts of success and failure. It is the pure joy of finding genuine fulfillment in your activities. Instead of losing interest your work takes on new significance because you now have a *total* rather than a fragmented perspective; this change is usually dramatically reflected in the quality of what you produce. In addition, if you are emitting vibrations of contentment in your work, you will find that the most remarkable resolutions take place in problems of relationships that may exist in your working environment.

I am well aware, I assure you, of the difficulty of making the above concepts crystal clear to your intellect. But this is not my objective. I am not concerned with your gaining a thorough intellectual grasp of the concept of nonattachment, loss of ego, "letting go," because in the final analysis you come to realize that these things have nothing to do with an "understanding" by your intellectual faculties; they have to do with *an experience by your total being.* Nonattachment is not understood; it is experienced. In essence what I am stating here, in an interpretation of the ancient wisdom of *Karma* Yoga and the *Bhagavad Gita,* is that many of the major problems that are connected with your work occur because the ego, the I, perpetuates continual needs and desires that are not, in fact, those of your true self. The dissolution of the ego, even for a few minutes at a time, results in an entirely different attitude and approach toward your work. Remember that we are speaking of an experience, and because it is an experience of the most profound nature, no amount of writing can truly convey what is involved. What I hope to accomplish with this discussion is to touch that center in you that is receptive to the wisdom of *Karma* Yoga; then you will realize the efficacy of experimenting with its principles. These principles can be applied on the job, like an exercise, as often as you can remember to do so. They are applicable even in the midst of your most demanding tasks. Similar to our physical exercises, this practice is progressive: as you gain mastery of the techniques, there is a corresponding evolution of your consciousness. Specifically, you are attempting to transcend the ego through the continual dedication of your work efforts to a higher principle; complete absorbtion in your work so that you *become* your work, your work flows through you; the conscious attempt to attain a state of nonattachment to the fruits of your labors, whatever these fruits may be.

The application of these *Karma* Yoga principles will be just as meaningful to those whose work would appear to present a minimum of the problems we listed at the beginning of this discussion. Artists, writers, musicians and composers, doctors, teachers, those connected with religious or service organizations may seem more fortunate in that their work is interesting, satisfying, and compensating. But with reflection these people may well discover that ultimate fulfillment in their work is being inhibited by the formidable intercedence of the ego. Actually, it is just these professions that require the least possible imposition of the ego and in which it often has its strongest hold. At my lectures on this subject students will often raise this objection: "But the ego is the thing that is responsible for the creative person's individual style; without the ego there will be no self-expression." On the contrary, it is only at those times when the ego is truly transcended, when the sense of an individual "I" can be dissolved, that an original "style" emerges and genuine self-expression is experienced. It is the egoless state that permits the greatest receptivity to the creative current and in which all truly creative people execute their most significant work.

Let me conclude this section by stating that I have never yet met a person who is seriously applying the principles of *Karma* Yoga who does not find himself in harmony with his work and who does not feel that his work is an indispensable part of his life. You, too, as a *Karma* Yogi will either achieve this harmony with your present work or, in keeping with the immutable laws of metaphysics, find that work which *is* in concert with your abilities and requirements gravitates toward you.

Reflecting on these principles is an excellent way to occupy your mind, whenever possible, on your way to work. Such elevating prework thoughts will usually be far more conducive to a productive and satisfying day than reading the newspaper, small talk with fellow commuters, or allowing the mind to engage in its endless fantasies without purpose.

A.M. "BREAK"
(a 5 minute routine)

Having discussed the application of the *Karma* Yoga principles, we can now learn how to use the *Hatha* Yoga techniques to very great advantage while on the job.

I strongly advocate that brief intervals of time be taken during working hours to relieve physical and emotional tensions, replenish vitality, and clear the mind. These are necessary not only for your health and well-being but for maintaining your job efficiency. There are several groups of Yoga exercises that provide perfect revitalizing methods. Most jobs afford a morning and afternoon "break" during which these routines can be performed. If you are self-employed, if you work at home, if you have your own office, you can probably break whenever you wish. If your break is at a prescribed time on your job, you should establish the habit of using five minutes of it for these revitalizing routines. The exercises consist primarily of very simple but effective stretching movements and with one exception can be done in your chair without leaving your desk.

Some of my students to whom I taught these on-the-job routines initially expressed concern about being conspicuous and drawing unwanted attention. But subsequently a number found they were able to get off by themselves; others reported that after a few days the novelty wore off for their fellow employees and what they were doing was simply accepted without further question; in many instances students were soon joined by their co-workers; still others told me that the routines are so beneficial they have grown oblivious to what others may think or say. It's interesting to note in this connection that a number

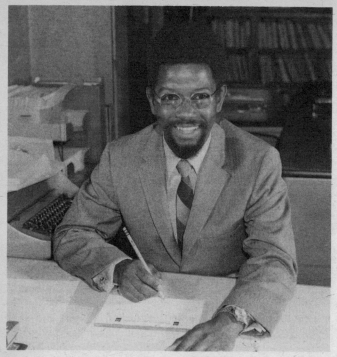

Jonathan Lee has been attending our Yoga classes for four months. He is the employment counselor at a large high school and is also involved in projects dealing with the social problems of his community. He intends to introduce the Yoga practice as a form of therapy for certain of these problems.

of companies recently initiated a voluntary "exercise break," having determined that such a program increases efficiency and decreases absenteeism.

I spend a good part of my day writing my books and programs; when I feel tension building and my mind becoming dull, I stop work and revitalize myself with the routines presented in this book under "A.M. and P.M. Break." These routines have evolved from a great deal of experimenting, and I present the exercises exactly as I do them. I'm sure you will find the routines as valuable as I have.

CHEST EXPANSION
(2 minutes)

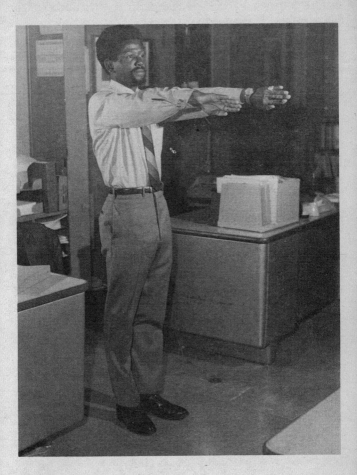

FIG. 26

In a standing position, with your heels together, slowly and gracefully bring your arms up from your sides into the position illustrated. Make sure to feel your elbows stretching (to remove tension).

FIG. 27

Slowly and gracefully bring your arms straight back on a line with your shoulders and clasp your hands as high as possible. Do not bend forward.

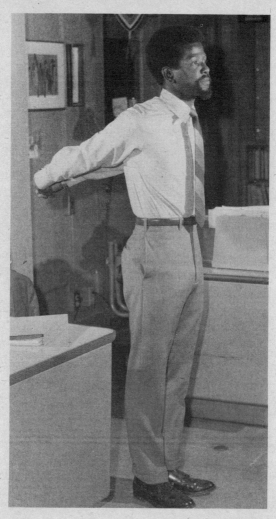

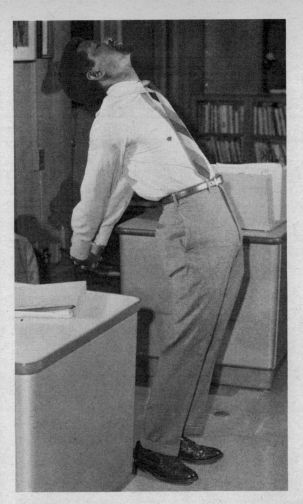

FIG. 28

Keep your arms raised as high as possible (for the shoulders). Very slowly, gently, and cautiously bend backward at the waist a moderate distance (for the spine). Arms must remain high, knees do not bend, head is back.

Count a slow 5.

FIG. 29

Now very slowly bend forward as far as possible without strain (also for the spine). Arms are held high, head is down, neck relaxed (let the blood flow into the brain). Hold motionless and count a slow 10.

FIG. 30

A more advanced position that will come naturally as your spine gains elasticity.

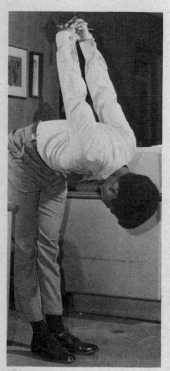
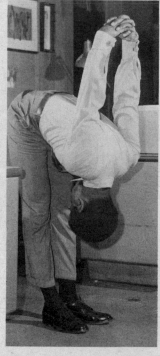

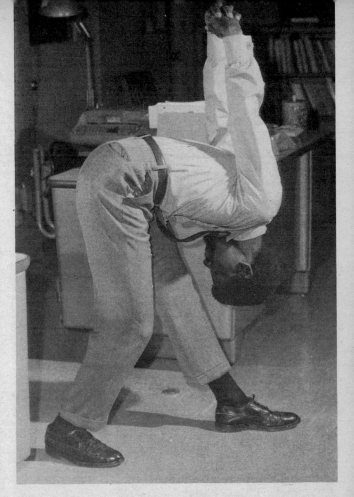

FIG. 31

Now, to stretch away tensions that accumulate in the knees and thighs, straighten up slightly so that you can extend your left leg out to the side as illustrated. Bend forward slowly as before, but now aim your forehead toward your left knee. Bend your right knee slightly to aid in the stretch.

Hold for 10.

FIG. 32

Straighten up slightly so that you can draw your left leg in and extend your right. Perform the same movements to the right knee.

Hold for 10.

Slowly straighten to the upright position; draw your right leg in, unclasp your hands, and relax a few moments without movement.

Repeat the entire routine once.

This one exercise stretches away tensions in the elbows, shoulders, spine, legs, and brings additional blood into the head for the eyes and brain.

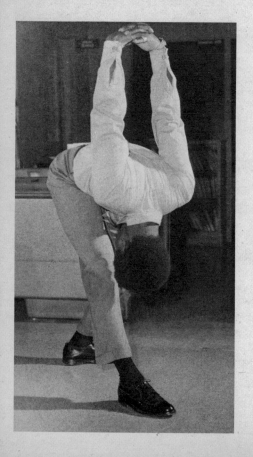

HEAD TWIST
(1 minute)

The neck is also a point where acute tension is continually accumulating. Here is one of two exercises we perform specifically to remove this tension.

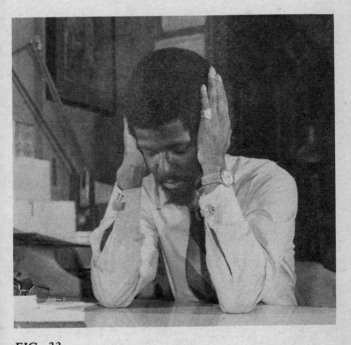

FIG. 33

Sit in your chair. Position your elbows close together on your desk and place your head between your hands. Close your eyes.

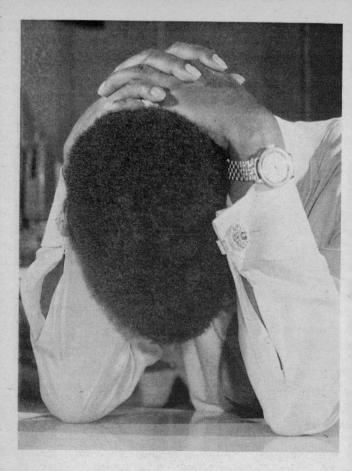

FIG. 34

Clasp your hands on the lower back of your head. Very slowly and gently push your head down until your chin touches your chest.

Hold for 20.

FIG. 35

Do not move your arms. Turn your head very slowly and rest your chin in your left hand. Grip the back of your head firmly with your right hand. Very, very slowly, with the aid of your hands, turn your head as far as possible to the left. Keep your eyes closed.

Hold for 20.

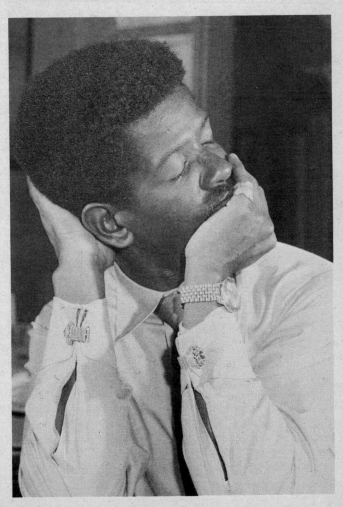

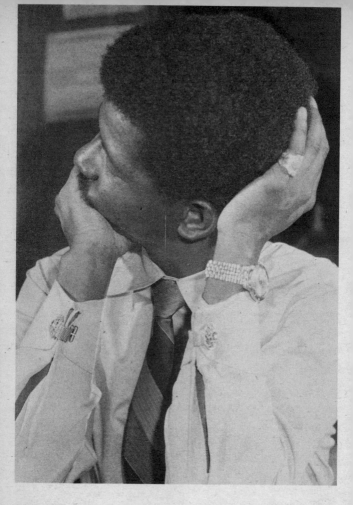

FIG. 36

Do not move your arms. Perform the same movements to the right side. Hold for 20. (When you have turned your head as far as possible without strain, you can probably go an extra cautious inch with the aid of a little extra pressure by your hands.)

Perform only once.

SIMPLE SPINAL TWIST
(1 minute)

This is a series of movements that releases and gives you access to energy that is locked in the spine.

FIG. 37
Seated in a chair, cross your right leg over the left.

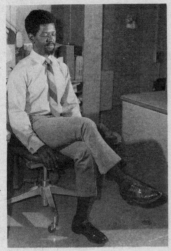

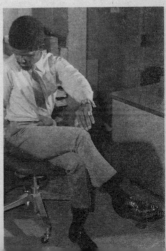

FIG. 38

Grip the back of the seat of the chair with your right hand. Cross your left arm *over* your right knee and take a firm hold of your left knee. This movement locks the lumbar area against which we can now twist the upper spine.

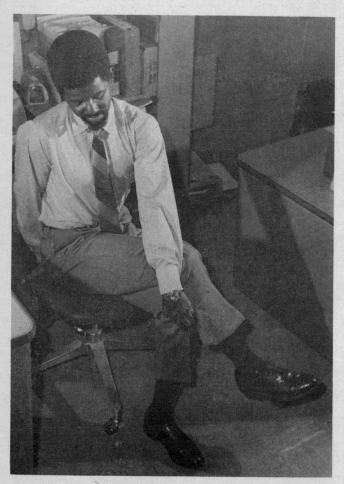

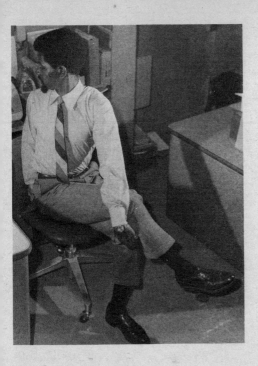

FIG. 40

Gripping the seat of the chair and holding your left knee firmly, *very slowly* twist your head and trunk as far as possible to the *right*. Be sure that your head, not only your trunk, is turned.

Hold without motion for 10.

Very slowly turn the head and trunk to the original frontward position but continue to hold the chair and your knee.

Relax a moment.

Repeat once.

Now cross the left leg over the right and perform the identical movements, twisting to the left side twice.

Note the instantaneous loosening as well as revitalizing properties of this exercise.

BACK STRETCH
(1 minute)

FIG. 41

Sit toward the edge of your chair. Extend your legs outward as illustrated. Bend forward and hold your upper calves firmly.

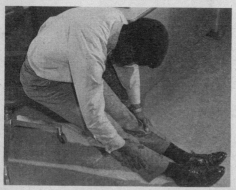

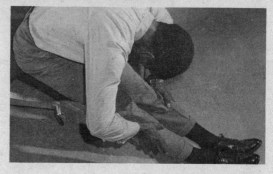

FIG. 42

Bend your elbows outward and very slowly and gently pull your trunk down. Relax all muscles, including those of your neck, so that your head hangs down (this is simply a stretch and there is no need to be tense in any area).

Hold without motion for a count of 20.

Very slowly straighten up and rest a moment.

FIG. 43

Now reach forward and down farther, as far as the lower calves or the ankles if possible, and execute the identical movements.

Hold for 20.

Slowly straighten up and rest.

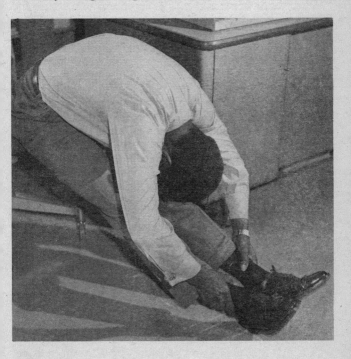

This completes the five minute routine. You will now find yourself pleasantly relaxed. However, this is also a *revitalizing* routine of a delayed nature: about fifteen minutes after returning to your work you will realize that you feel energized, your mind more alert. I have suggested to my students who hold various executive positions that they perform the above five minute routine about fifteen minutes prior to any important business meeting. If you try this once, the reasons for my suggestion will be obvious.

FOR THE HOUSEWIFE

Since the housewife spends a significant part of her life in housework this work must also be, from the Yogic viewpoint, meaningful. It has been my experience with students who are housewives that they do find an overall fulfillment in providing their families with the necessities of domestic life. However, the major obstacle that the housewife encounters is the sameness of her work, the monotony of those chores that must be repeated over and over again on a daily basis. It is certainly difficult to speak about "sustaining one's interest" in these tasks, and yet we find if the housewife keeps in satisfactory physical and psychological condition, if her energy is adequate and her spirits good, she can not only perform these repetitious chores without a sense of drudgery but also cope with the pressures and responsibilities that other aspects of being a wife and mother require.

The housewife can help herself enormously by taking a midmorning and midafternoon break during her work-day to keep herself physically and mentally fit. She may say, "But I exercise all day—cleaning, sweeping, washing, shopping, gardening, keeping up with the children—it's all exercise." Definitely not. It's movement, and perhaps a great deal of movement, but it's not exercise. Genuine exercise, for our purposes, is *methodical manipulation of the body.* Most of the work activities in which the house-wife is involved create and promote stress, strain, tension. Our Yoga movements, especially those of the "break" routines, reduce and eliminate these conditions; they act to minimize fatigue, irritation, and depression.

In addition to the five minute routine in the preceding pages, the housewife can take an extra few minutes and do the two exercises that follow. These will firm and streamline her body and impart grace, poise, and balance, all very important in maintaining her self-confidence and good spirits.

DANCER'S EXERCISE
(2 minutes)

FIG. 44*

In a standing position with your feet slightly apart, place your palms together and rest your hands on the top of your head. Note the symmetry of the arms.

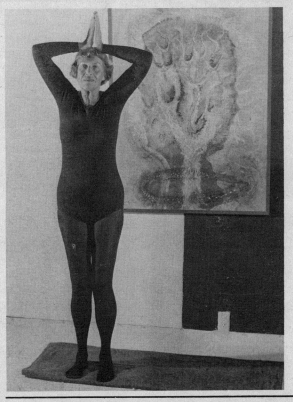

* Our model for this and several other exercises that appear in the book is Louisa Jenkins, an excellent Yoga student and noted artist. She was photographed in her studio and home, taking a few minutes from her work for a Yoga break. She is 73 years old.

FIG. 45

In very slow motion bend your knees and lower your body as far as possible.

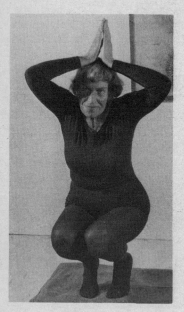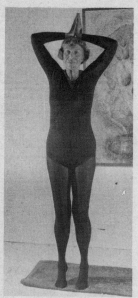

FIG. 46

Without pause begin to push up very slowly, remaining on your toes all the way up until you are in the position illustrated. Then rest your soles on the floor and repeat without pause.

Perform 10 times in continuous slow motion. There are no pauses in this exercise.

Remember to move as slowly as possible. If you lose your balance at any point, stop completely; regain your balance and your composure and proceed from where you were or start over. Do not laugh at yourself if a loss of balance occurs. The Dancer's Exercise will firm and strengthen your legs and help you gain a good sense of balance that will be reflected in your carriage.

CIRCULAR MOTION
(3 minutes)

*FIG. 47**

Stand erect with your feet together and your hands on your hips. Bend forward slightly as illustrated.

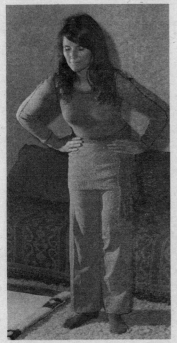

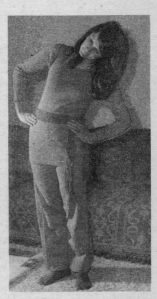

FIG. 48

Slowly roll and twist in a small circle to your left. Keep your knees straight and do not move your legs. Only the trunk rolls and twists.

Hold the position without movement for a count of 2.

---

* Our model for a number of the exercises, including two of the more difficult "balance" postures, is Lore Kuhns, principal instructor at the Yoga for Health Center in Carmel, California.

FIG. 49
Slowly roll and twist your trunk in a small circle to the backward position.

Hold for 2.

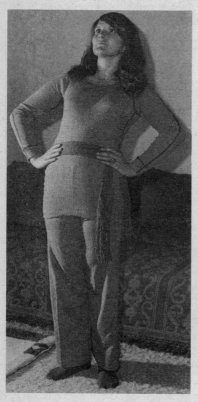
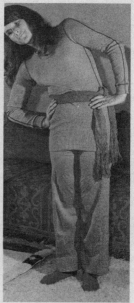

FIG. 50

Slowly roll and twist in a small circle to your right.

Hold for 2.

Slowly roll and twist in a small circle to the original frontward position.

Hold for 2.

FIG. 51

Now bend forward several inches further than when you began. Compare Figs. 51 and 47.

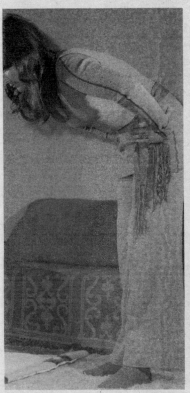
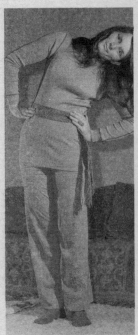

FIG. 52

The object now is to make a wider circle with your trunk. Slowly roll and twist in a wider (intermediate) circle to your left. Compare Figs. 52 and 48.

Continue the wider circle with the trunk by rolling and twisting first to the backward position and then to the right.

Hold each for a count of 2.

Roll and twist to the frontward position of Fig. 51.

FIG. 53
The object now is to make the widest circle possible without strain. Bend forward as far as possible.

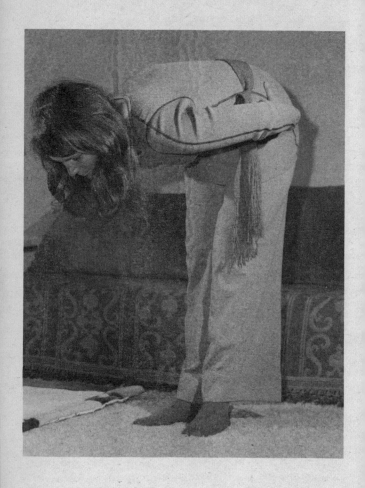

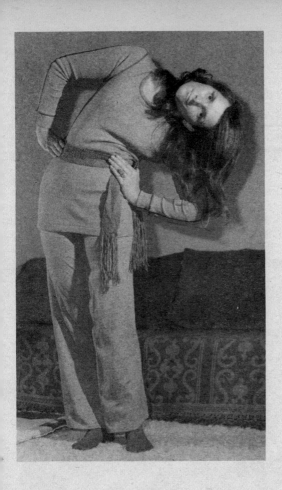

FIG. 54

Roll and twist as far as possible to your left. Compare with Fig. 52.

Continue the widest circle possible by rolling and twisting to the backward, right, and forward positions.

Hold each for a rhythmic count of 2.

When you have completed the movements, straighten up and rest a few moments.

Repeat the identical movements from each of the 3 positions. Perform the entire routine from each of the 3 positions 5 times. If you are seriously attempting to reduce the waist and hips, you can do as many as 10 rounds. Perform the movements rhythmically, pausing in each position for a count of 2. Keep the image of making the widening circles as you roll and twist your trunk.

Very important: this is not a series of simple bends. The movements are intensive *rolls and twists* with exaggerated action in the waist and hips.

There are many exercise-type movements that can be incorporated into your housework. One of my students who had really perfected these movements brought a broom to class and at her request we obtained a vacuum cleaner from our janitor. She demonstrated the long, graceful movements that can be performed while using these implements. In her hands they became more like dancing partners than a broom and vacuum cleaner. She also showed how she made a kind of dance out of straightening up a room. My main point is that if poise and balance are kept firmly in mind, your body will respond accordingly and a number of the "drudgery" chores can turn into fun and beneficial exercise!

SNACKS

(See the section on "Nutrition")

LUNCHTIME

Most working people have only a brief interval for lunch, and in addition to eating in whatever time is allotted, they will often attempt to accomplish other tasks including shopping. So lunchtime is usually very social (lunch is eaten with friends) and often very busy, even frantic. To speak about exercising or giving thoughts to self-improvement during this interval may seem thoroughly impractical. But it frequently happens that people who begin to practice Yoga find their approach to many activities changing. "Getting with yourself" seems to become one of the most rewarding endeavors of life, and you may feel that it is necessary to gain additional time for increased introspection. In this event you will find yourself automatically becoming less involved in activities that seem to pull you into the world of objects and superfluous relationships, things that drain your life force and prevent your consciousness from expanding. It will then become important to you to set aside at least a few minutes during your lunchtime to reflect on some of the philosophic principles we have previously discussed that relate to work and even to utilize one or two of the physical techniques.

In my travels I held over one hundred jobs consisting of many different types of work. In each and every one of these I found it absolutely essential to get off by myself for a few minutes at lunchtime so that I might maintain my perspective. These few minutes proved invaluable for reinforcing the Yogic principles, the inner work in which I was involved. So I speak again from experience when I make this suggestion: eat your lunch with your friends or business associates if you wish; do your shopping or whatever you must; but save five to ten minutes to be alone, to either sit down and withdraw your thoughts from the outer world for a brief period of reflection or to take a short walk in conjunction with performing the Complete Breath. The latter would be done as follows: as you walk in a fairly brisk manner, you perform the abdominal and chest (not the shoulder) movements of the Complete Breath. Since these movements are inconspicuous you need not be concerned about drawing attention to yourself. The breathing is *continuous;* unlike the Complete Breath of our "Arising" routine *there is no holding of the breath;* each breath flows directly into the next. If you walk for five to ten minutes you can do at least twenty-five Complete Breaths. In concentrating fully on the movements your thoughts will be directed inward, and you will return to work refreshed and strengthened rather than drained. In the course of my own jobs I have done this walking-breathing exercise in many different places: on city streets, in parks, on quiet roads, on railroad tracks, and I even devised ways of walking indoors during inclement weather. The technique is always effective regardless of where it's done.

LUNCH

(See the section on "Nutrition")

P.M. "BREAK"
(a 5 minute routine)

The afternoon "break" routine can be done in its entirety without leaving your chair. Here again a group of simple movements performed exactly as instructed are able to reach into tension areas, relieve fatigue, replenish energy, and help clear the mind.

FINGER EXERCISE
(15 seconds)

As the day progresses there is a definite build-up of tension in the fingers. This can be relieved through simple stretching.

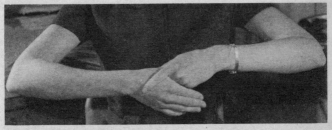

FIG. 55

Hold the thumb of the right hand firmly, as far down as possible. Pull quite hard and hold the pull for a count of 2.

Next pull on the index finger and hold for a count of 2.

Pull on each of the remaining three fingers in turn.

FIG. 56

Perform the identical movements with the fingers of the left hand. Once with each finger is sufficient.

The Yoga routines manipulate every part of the body. The fingers must not be neglected (especially if you note regular stiffness or any signs of arthritis).

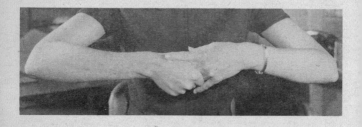

ELBOW EXERCISE
(15 seconds)

Another area that is seldom consciously exercised is the elbows. During our morning break routine we stretched the elbows in the Chest Expansion exercise. Now we concentrate on them with a different type of movement.

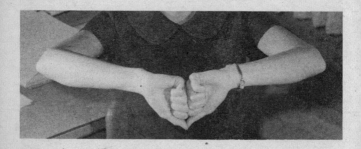

FIG. 57

Make fists of your hands and raise your arms to the position depicted. The elbows are bent and the backs of the hands are drawn in toward you.

FIG. 58

In one of the few quick movements we perform in Yoga, the arms are quickly and forcefully snapped outward. The joints of the elbows will often "crack" in this movement, indicating a desirable loosening. Hold the arms straight for a moment, then bend the elbows once again and repeat.

Perform 10 times.

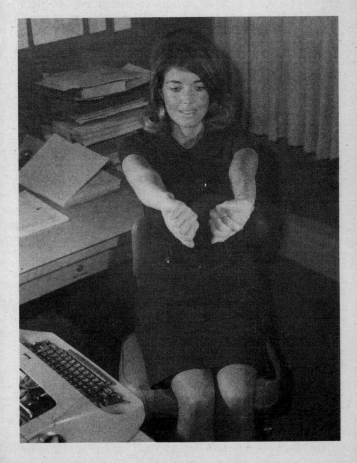

MOVEMENTS FOR THE SHOULDERS AND NECK

The shoulders and neck are two of the most severe tension points in the entire body; tightness and stiffness in the muscles of these areas are frequently present without our knowledge and can be responsible for fatigue and a continual vague discomfort. This is particularly true if you spend a significant amount of time sitting at a desk. We therefore do well to manipulate the shoulders and neck in the morning (with the Chest Expansion and Head Twist) and now in the afternoon with the following three exercises.

SHOULDER RAISE
(30 seconds)

You will require sufficient room to extend your arms straight outward behind you.

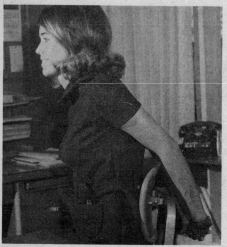

FIG. 59
Interlace your fingers behind you.

FIG. 60

In very slow motion raise your arms as high as possible without strain. Straighten the elbows if you can. Keep your spine straight, don't bend forward. Feel the shoulders being stretched.

Hold your extreme position without motion for 5.

Very slowly lower your arms. Rest a moment.

Perform 3 times very slowly.

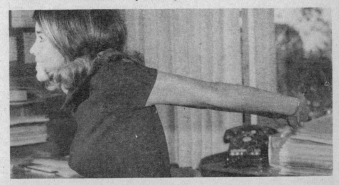

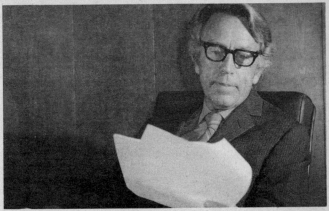

Frank Riley is the manager of a large cultural and recreatonal center. He has been practicing Yoga for only one month, and although he is able to devote a minimum of time he has made excellent progress in the routines and is finding them, in his own words, "Extremely helpful in the intellectual and emotional areas."

POSTURE CLASP
(1 minute)

This exercise is also primarily for the shoulders. It manipulates them differently than the previous set of movements. People who are "round-shouldered" or who are developing a "dowager's hump" will find this exercise helpful.

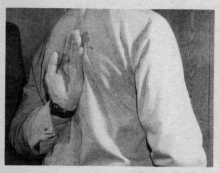

FIG. 61
Position yourself in your chair so that you can bring your left arm up as illustrated. The palm faces away from your back. Sit erect.

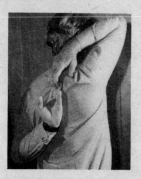

FIG. 62
Bring your right hand over and lock your fingers.

FIG. 63

Very slowly and gently pull up with your right arm so that the left arm is raised 1 or 2 inches. Sit erect, don't slump.

Hold for 5.

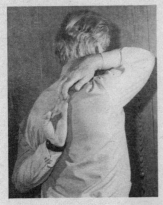

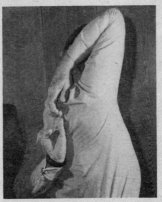

FIG. 64

Slowly and gently pull down with your left arm so that the right is lowered 1 or 2 inches. Remain erect.

Hold for 5.

Repeat these up and down pulls once more.

FIG. 65
Reverse the position of the arms. **Perform the up and down pulls twice, as before. Unclasp the hands and relax briefly.**

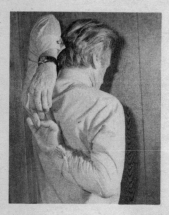

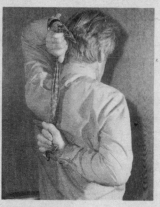

FIG. 66

You may experience some difficulty at first in having the hands meet behind you. Usually, this becomes possible with a few days of practice. If not, hold a handkerchief, piece of cloth, or towel and execute the pulling movements while holding this material.

HEAD ROLL
(1 minute, 15 seconds)

In the morning break routine we manipulated the head with our hands. This exercise, which requires a different type of movement, is equally effective and extremely relaxing.

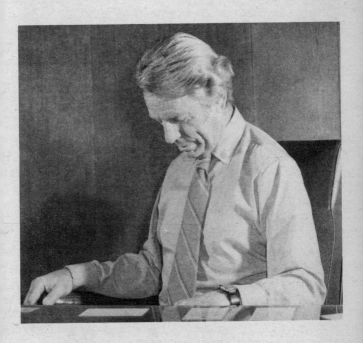

FIG. 67

If you're wearing glasses, remove them. Close your eyes. Slowly bend your head forward and allow your chin to rest on your chest.

Hold without motion for a count of 5.

FIG. 68

In very slow motion roll and twist your head to the extreme left. Don't just bend your head to the side; it rolls and twists in a slow, even exaggerated motion. Keep your eyes closed.

Hold for 5.

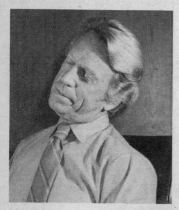

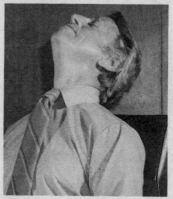

FIG. 69

In very slow motion roll and twist your head to the extreme backward position. Feel your chin and throat stretching.

Hold for 5.

FIG. 70

In very slow motion roll and twist your head to the extreme right. Eyes remain closed.

Hold for 5.

In very slow motion roll and twist your head to the original frontward position.

Hold for 5.

Perform the entire routine 3 times in extremely slow motion. If you are prone to severe tension in your neck, repeat several additional times.

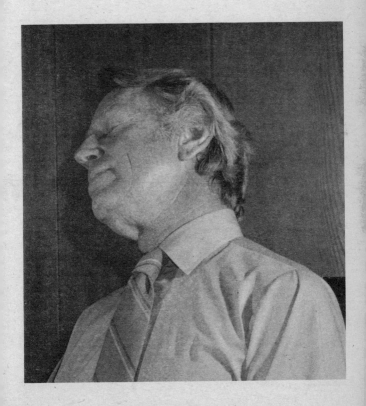

EYE EXERCISE
(1 minute, 45 seconds)

We all treasure our sight, and yet how many people do you know who take the time to exercise their eyes? In my beginning classes when I ask students how many of them brush their teeth, all hands are raised. But when I ask them about eye care, I find that less than one in 50 has ever exercised his eyes! The following movements, requiring less than two minutes, will provide effective exercise for these vital organs.

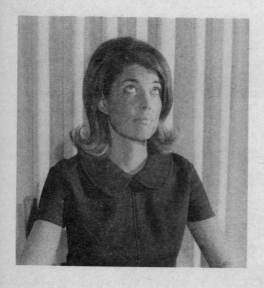

FIG. 71

If you wear glasses you should have already removed them for the previous exercise.

Widen your eye sockets and hold them wide throughout this exercise. Move your eyes slowly to the top of the sockets.

Hold 1 second.

FIG. 72

Slowly roll your eyes to the extreme left. Do it slowly and make the muscles work. Keep the sockets wide.

Hold 1 second. (This is not a continuous rolling of the eyes.)

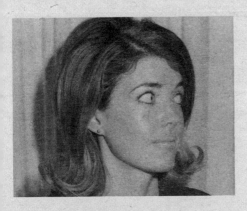

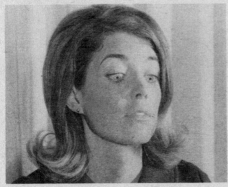

FIG. 73

Slowly roll your eyes to the extreme bottom. Keep the sockets wide. (This wide position helps to remove tension in the muscles around the eyes.)

Hold 1 second.

FIG. 74

Slowly roll your eyes to the extreme right.

Hold 1 second.

Repeat this routine of the 4 positions and perform 10 times in all. The eyes move slowly and rhythmically and you must feel that the muscles are getting a workout by moving to the extreme positions in the sockets.

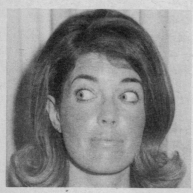

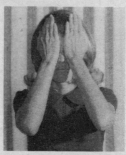

FIG. 75

Now close your eyes and place your palms over them as depicted. Hold for a minimum count of 30. Turn your mind inward and attempt to hold it "thoughtless" for this brief interval.

This completes the 5 minute routine.

FOR THE HOUSEWIFE

Again, for the housewife, or those who are working in a more leisurely or private situation and who want to spend a few extra minutes in figure improvement, we offer the following two Yoga exercises. These are to be performed *in addition* to the preceding routine.

TRIANGLE
(2 minutes, 30 seconds)

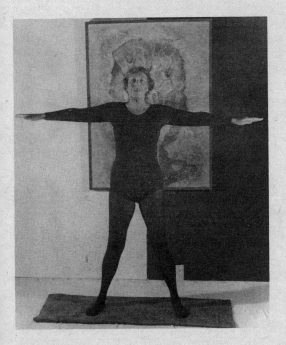

FIG. 76
Assume the position illustrated. Note that your palms face downward and your legs are in a moderately wide stance.

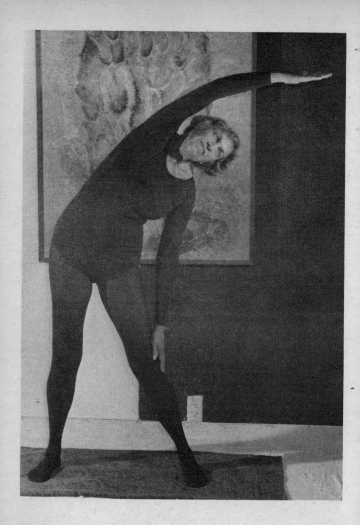

FIG. 77

Slowly bend your trunk to the left. Your left hand rests in the area of your left knee and your right arm is brought over your head into the position illustrated, palm facing downward. Knees remain straight.

108

FIG. 78

Now *very slowly* continue to bring your right arm over and down until it is parallel with the floor. You must do this lowering of the arm very slowly so that you can feel the tightening and firming on your right side.

Hold without motion for 10.

Slowly straighten up and perform the identical movements on the right side.

Repeat the same movements, first to the left, then to the right. The legs remain in their original position.

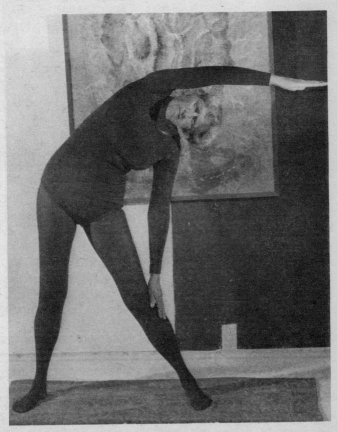

FIG. 79

Slowly straighten to the upright position and lower your arms. Now assume the widest possible stance. Compare this with Fig. 76.

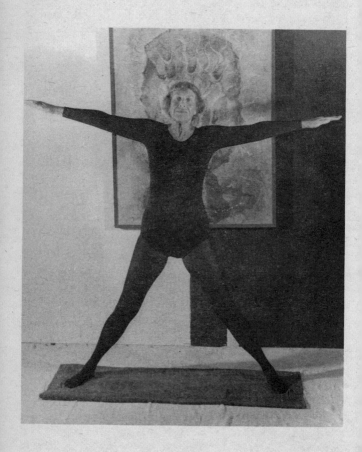

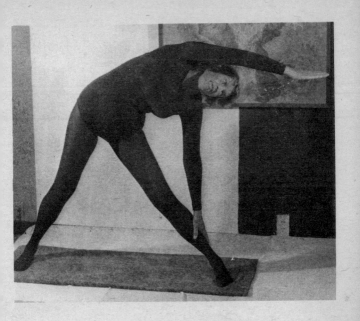

FIG. 80

The left hand holds the lower calf or ankle. The arm is slowly lowered, as before, to the parallel position. You will feel how this movement is able to tighten and firm the inside of your thighs in a most effective way.

Hold for 10.

Slowly straighten up and perform the identical movements on the right side.

Repeat the same movements once more, first to the left side, then to the right.

Slowly straighten to the upright position; slowly lower arms to sides; draw the legs together; relax a few moments.

This is an excellent exercise for helping to redistribute weight. (Note the triangles formed with the limbs in the extreme positions.)

ABOUT BALANCE

I place particular emphasis on the value of cultivating a good sense of balance. In my classes I go to great lengths to teach the Yoga balance exercises in detail, and I always make sure that each student is trying his very best to master them. Some students want to give up these exercises almost immediately, believing that if they do not succeed in their first attempts, they never will be able to do them properly. They seem to feel, "Either you have it or you don't." But I know that very good balance *can* be developed in almost everyone, and I strongly encourage this development because I have seen the most remarkable changes occur in the entire appearance of people who have not had good balance and who subsequently gain it.

All movement is related to balance and one's carriage, the way she (or he) holds herself, her style of walking, her poise, indeed, everything she does, from serving tea to playing tennis, is inestimably improved through a heightened sense of balance. It is one of the most important factors in figure improvement and an essential dynamic in what is referred to as the "mystique" of beauty; rhythmic flowing motions are attributes of true beauty, and characteristic of that person who is secure in her balance.

I urge you to make every effort to master the following exercise regardless of your age or any previous difficulty you may have had with balance. Actually, the patient and regular practice of these movements will go a long way toward imparting those desirable qualities mentioned above. In very short order the balance "awareness" will penetrate your consciousness, and you will find this reflected in the way you approach not only the Yoga exercises but just about everything you do.

BALANCE POSTURE
(2 minutes, 30 seconds)

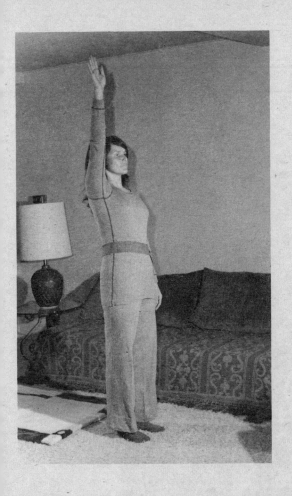

FIG. 81
In a standing position slowly raise your right arm straight overhead.

FIG. 82

Slowly raise your left leg behind you and hold your left foot with the left hand.

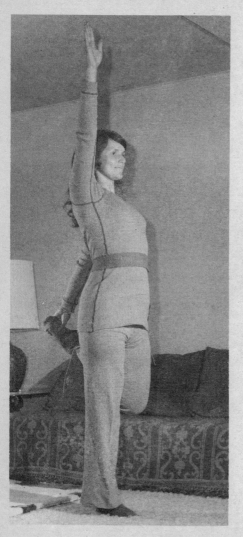

114

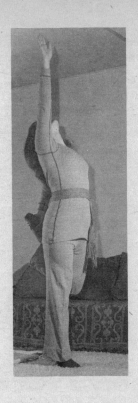

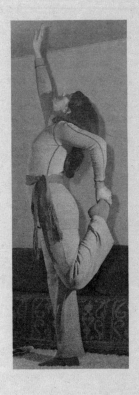

FIGS. 83A and 83B

Very slowly and cautiously bring your left foot up and your right arm back. Drop your head back. Hold as still as possible for 5.

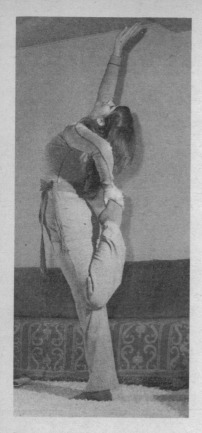

FIG. 84

The extreme position that you should perform once you are sure of your balance in the preceding position. The leg has now been drawn up as far as possible and the raised arm is back.

This extreme position is also held for 5.

Very slowly lower the arm and leg; rest a moment without fidgeting and perform the identical movements on the opposite side.

Perform 3 times on each side, alternating the sides, i.e., left-right, left-right, left-right.

FIG. 85

A variation that is to be considered as an advanced position and should be attempted only when you are very secure in Fig. 84. It is done directly following Fig. 84 without lowering the arm and leg; it is also held as still as possible for 5.

I can estimate that I have been witness to more than 25,000 losses of balance in this exercise, and it is highly probable that you, too, will lose your balance frequently during the course of practice. This is exactly what the learning process entails. When loss of balance occurs you must pause for a moment, regain your composure, and begin again. Each time you do this you will come closer to mastering the posture, and one day you'll find that you have it. In the beginning you will note that on some days you meet with much more success than on others. This, too, is natural in the learning process. In losing your balance you must *never laugh at yourself;* not even a smile. Maintain a very serious attitude and your progress will be accelerated.

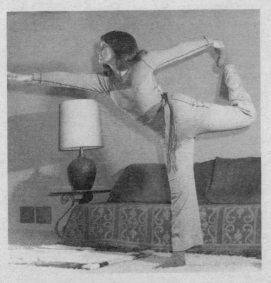

SNACKS

(See the section on "Nutrition")

RETURNING HOME
(a 10 minute routine)

The devitalizing nature of many jobs, coupled with what, for most commuters, is a harrowing trip home, usually results in a state of acute fatigue and irritability. The accepted homecoming remedies for this type of physical and emotional exhaustion include the complete collapse into one's chair, a nap, an alcoholic beverage or tranquilizing pill to induce artificial relaxation. A special ten minute Yoga routine can be more advantageous to your well-being and more effective for your overall enjoyment of the evening than any or all of the above.

If, to the uninitiated, self-improvement practices during lunchtime seemed highly questionable, serious exercising upon returning home from work would probably appear as the height of absurdity. "Why," they would ask, "would

we want to further tax our already exhausted bodies?"
Of course, those whom I speak of as "uninitiated" think of
exercising in terms of the usual quick, strenuous, repetitious movements of calisthenics. But if at this point, you
have tested some of our suggestions and routines you
fully realize that Yoga techniques are very different from
calisthenics. Yoga movements are nonstrenuous and are
performed easily and slowly to *increase* our vitality, release trapped energy, relieve tension, and restore our
emotional equilibrium. Since we now know that such
things can be accomplished in a way that is not only nonstrenuous but actually enjoyable (it feels good to stretch
deeply, to bring blood into tired areas, to clear the lungs
and brain through correct breathing), it makes very good
sense to spend ten minutes when we return home from
work in divesting ourselves of tensions, and preparing
ourselves to enjoy the evening. This latter is especially
important: if you come home tired, irritable, depressed
you seldom recover, and these negative conditions color
your entire evening. But if, as soon as possible after returning home, *before* you rest, drink, or eat, you perform
the following ten minute routine, within the hour you will
find yourself delightfully refreshed. For such results ten
minutes is not much time to spend, is it? However, let me
reiterate: it is essential that the routine be practiced as
soon as possible upon returning home, *before* you rest
or become involved in any activity. If you do the "break"
routines during the day, you will certainly reduce, to a
significant degree, the negative conditions of your workday; even so, due to many factors, you may return home
with tensions. Wash, either change into some loose clothing
suitable for stretching, or simply remove your shoes, belt,
watch, glasses, tie, take your Yoga mat, and try to get off
by yourself quietly for this ten minute routine. You can
rest, eat, drink, and so forth upon its completion.

Note to those who work at home: do the routine as
soon as possible following the end of your workday.

Note to housewives: do the routine late in the afternoon
before your husband comes home. If you go shopping in
the afternoon you'll probably come home tired. Do the
routine as soon as possible upon returning.

THE BACK AND SPINE

Before we begin the exercises of this routine it will probably be revealing for you to consider for a few moments the type of exercise your back receives during your workday. In one of my classes I selected six students with varied work activities: a typist, a salesman (in a clothing store), an elementary school teacher, a dentist, a construction worker, and a housewife. I asked each to observe, during the course of one workweek, the type of movements in which his (her) back was involved. This was done and in our next class the following week the six students gave us a demonstration of their primary back movements. The demonstration was extremely meaningful, not only to the six volunteers, but to the entire class of sixty-two students. We determined that: (1) in all sedentary jobs the back, is, for the most part, "frozen" into a very few positions (as was the case with the typist, salesman, and teacher, for although there was quite some body movement with the latter two, the back and spine themselves remained relatively rigid); (2) the type of work that required more movement and activity (the dentist and construction worker) seemed to cause a great deal of back stress and strain. Of the six, the one who had the most opportunity actually to exercise the back while "on the job" was the housewife (we have made some suggestions regarding the possibilities of doing just this in the "A.M. Break" section). The obvious conclusion was that very few jobs permit or encourage healthful movements for the back and spine. If you have ever examined the structure of the back, or have any knowledge of the way in which the spine functions, you can appreciate the necessity of regular, methodical manipulation for both. Since we can be fairly certain that your work does not involve such manipulation, it is obvious that you must take a few minutes for such practice at some point during the day; the most efficacious time is when you return home from work or shopping and back tensions are usually at their peak.

Of the tangible, real physical complaints of all people in the Western world, those pertaining to the back seem to head the list. There are very few families in which someone is not suffering from back trouble. Again, if you have even a partial understanding of the structures of the back and spine, you know how easily you can pull a muscle or damage a vertebra. I maintain (and all Yoga students will readily agree) that if the back is kept strong and the spine supple, you greatly improve your chances of *preventing* these troubles.

Also, Yoga has had a most salutary effect on all types of back conditions. I can cite dozens of dramatic instances. One that comes immediately to mind is that of Mr. George Stanicci, an architect and designer who resides in Los Angeles. Due to a back injury he walked in a severely stooped fashion, and when he first came to my Yoga classes he had been unable to straighten up for several years. He continually experienced the most acute discomfort. After approximately six months of cautious, intelligent Yoga practice all traces of his condition completely disappeared! Today he walks as straight as an arrow, and since discomfort is no longer written on his face he looks ten years younger. If you suffer from back trouble, Yoga may be the answer. Make sure that you receive your doctor's approval first, and then proceed very cautiously, following all my instructions to the letter.

The Yoga back exercises are extremely powerful; don't be deceived by their apparent simplicity. The movements reach deep into the muscles and vertebrae, and different exercises enable you to emphasize different areas: the lumbar, dorsals, and cervical. Once you become sensitive to how the various exercises affect you personally, you can devote additional time to those that pertain to your condition.

There are two excellent back exercises in this particular routine. The first works the spine concavely, the second convexly. (The Cobra and Full Twist exercises that appear in later routines are also important back exercises.)

BACK STRETCH
(1 minute, 30 seconds)

We have done a modified form of this exercise while seated in a chair during our "A.M. Break" routine. Now we perform the complete exercise in its classical form.

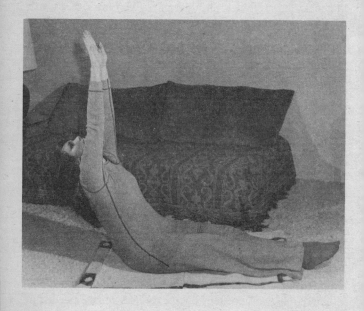

FIG. 86
Seated on your mat, stretch your legs straight out and keep your feet together. In very slow, graceful motion bring your arms up overhead and lean backward a few inches (to help tone your abdominal muscles).

FIG. 87
Rock your trunk gently from side to side (to loosen your spine) as you stretch forward, arms extended.

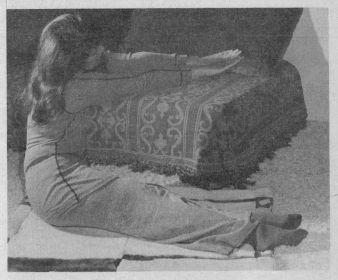

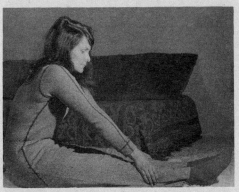

FIG. 88
Take a firm hold of your calves.

FIG. 89

Bend your elbows outward and very slowly and gently pull your trunk forward so that your head comes as close to your knees as possible. Head is down, neck relaxed. Make sure your elbows are bent as illustrated. Do not strain.

Hold without motion for 20.

Slowly straighten up, simultaneously bringing your arms into the extended position.

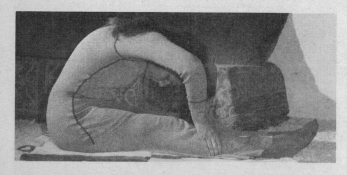

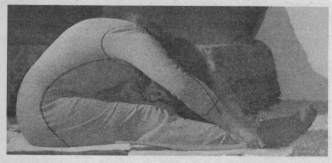

FIG. 90

Lean backward with your arms extended and perform the same movements, this time attempting to hold your ankles. If you cannot hold the ankles comfortably, revert to holding the calves.

Hold for 20.

FIG. 91

This advanced posture will be attained as your spine gains flexibility. The soles of the feet are held and the head rests on the knees. An intensive stretch, but not a strain, is experienced. Revert to the ankles if you feel any discomfort in this position. (Learn to distinguish between stretching and straining.) Hold for 20.

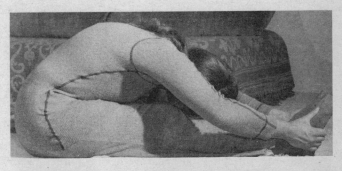

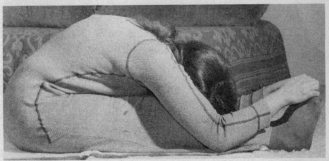

FIG. 92

This ultimate stretch is a continuation of Fig. 91. When you have eventually accomplished the position of Fig. 91 (and accomplish it you will), you will require even more of a challenge. Therefore, move the hands from the soles of the feet upward to hold the toes and drop the elbows down to touch the floor. Be very careful not to strain.

This is also held for 20.

Summary: this exercise should be done 3 times as follows: once to the calves, once to the ankles, once to your most extreme position. If you cannot hold the feet or toes, then you do 2 to the ankles. If you cannot hold the ankles, then you simply do 3 to the calves. Remember, 3 times; hold each stretch for 20. Even when you accomplish the extreme positions, you always do the calves and ankles also. Each is essential and none must be neglected because the various postures place emphasis on the different areas of the back and spine. This will be obvious to you if you concentrate fully on the movements as has been repeatedly urged in this text.

Beginning class students who see us perform the postures depicted in Figs. 91 and 92 are sometimes quick to exclaim, "I'll never be able to do that!" They are not yet aware of the body's ability to gain an astonishing degree of flexibility when subjected to the Yoga techniques. However, within a short time this flexibility begins to manifest and the student realizes how his spine was formerly compressed, the vertebrae pushed together. Nature is with you in these movements and will assist you in every way; you are not engaging in hostilities with your body when you practice Yoga. So reserve judgment on your ability in this or any of the Yoga exercises until you have practiced for a few weeks.

In this Back Stretch exercise the object is not to see how fast you can fight your way down. Never strain or jerk; simply hold the various areas of the legs according to your ability. There is no trick or shortcut to achieving the more extreme positions; this will happen progressively, naturally, as you gain flexibility.

BOW
(1 minute)

FIG. 93

Lie down gracefully and rest your chin on the mat. Reach back and hold your feet. (In the beginning you may have to struggle a few minutes to do this. Hold one foot first, then take hold of the other.)

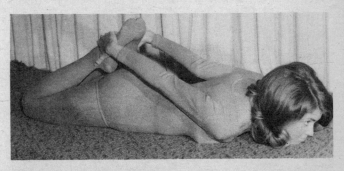

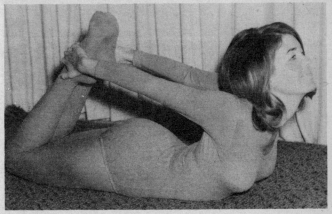

FIG. 94

Hold your feet firmly and very slowly and cautiously raise your trunk. Keep your head back.

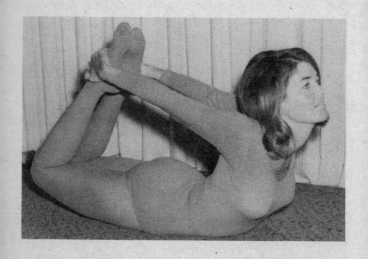

FIG. 95

Keep your trunk raised and slowly and cautiously raise your knees. Try to hold the knees together. Keep your head up and back. If you cannot raise your knees, simply hold your trunk up.

Hold for 10.

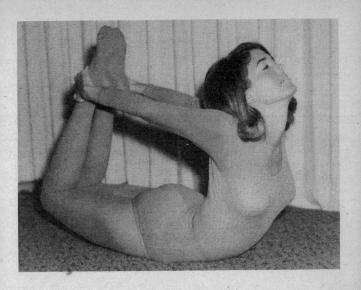

FIG. 96

The extreme position. Your trunk and knees are raised as high as possible (knees close together).

Hold whatever position you attain as motionless as possible for 10. It is important to come out of the posture as follows: first, slowly lower your knees to the floor but do not let go of your feet. Next, slowly lower your trunk and chin to the floor but continue to hold your feet. Finally, release the feet and slowly lower your legs to the floor.

Rest your cheek on the mat for a few moments and relax completely. Repeat once.

FIG. 97

If you are unable to hold your feet, loop hand towels or any material around them and attempt the raise with this aid.

This is a powerful toning and strengthening exercise for the back (as well as the thighs and chest), and the movements must be done as slowly and cautiously as indicated in the above instructions. Holding your knees together is preferable but, in the beginning, not essential. Practice to make the movements smooth. Never jerk or make any erratic movements in this exercise.

In the extreme position of Fig. 96 the body resembles the archer's bow.

You may have seen me instruct Art Linkletter in this exercise when I was a guest on his program. He did remarkably well in his very first attempt. Don't be in a hurry; you will succeed with practice.

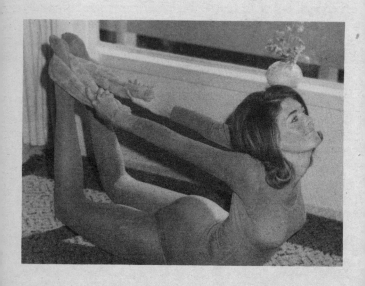

Since our next three Yoga exercises deal primarily with various areas of the legs, it is advisable to make a few comments about them here.

In connection with the housewife we stated that activity is often mistaken for exercise, the *amount* of movement being confused with the *type* of movement. This situation also pertains to people who are on their feet a great deal, taking many short walks in the course of their day's work. (These short distances can actually total several miles.) They are exhausted when they return home and believe that their legs have been thoroughly exercised. But it is not genuine exercise that has tired them. Long walks in rhythmic strides can be defined as "exercise," but many short walks in uneven tempos promote stress and fatigue.

On the other hand, weariness in the legs is also experienced by those who sit at their desks and do practically no walking at all during the day. Why? Because the muscles, which are not activated, stiffen, and because the blood flows continually downward into the legs without relief. So to counteract fatigue, tension, cramps in the legs two things are indicated: stretching and reversing the flow of the blood. The value of Yoga can again be appreciated when we realize it is possible to do the necessary exercises with a bare minimum of movement, making them ideal for the weary worker or housewife.

ALTERNATE LEG STRETCH
(2 minutes)

Stretching relieves tension and restores energy. This is an ingenious exercise that enables you to fully stretch the legs.

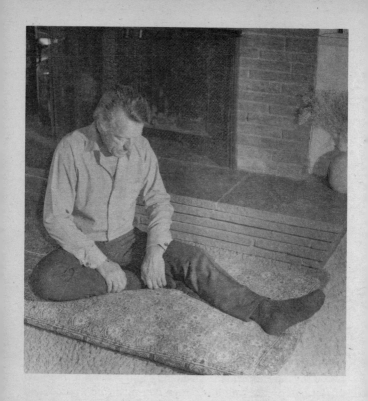

FIG. 98

Gracefully return to a sitting position with your legs extended. Place the sole of your right foot as high as possible against (not under) your left thigh.

FIG. 99
In very slow, graceful motion bring your arms up over-head and lean backward a few inches.

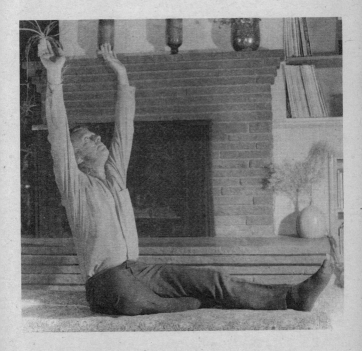

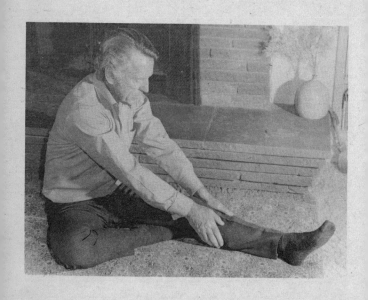

FIG. 100

Slowly reach forward and take a firm hold of your left calf.

FIG. 101

Bend your elbows outward and very slowly and gently pull your trunk forward so that your head comes as close to your left knee as possible. Head is down, neck relaxed.

Hold without motion for 10.

Slowly straighten up, simultaneously bringing your arms into the extended position overhead. Lean backward a few inches as before.

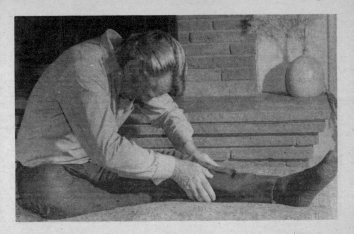

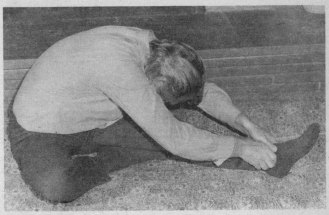

FIG. 102

Now stretch forward and attempt to hold the left ankle; perform the same stretching movements. If you cannot hold the ankle comfortably, revert to the calf.

Hold for 10.

Slowly straighten up with your arms extended as before. Lean backward.

135

FIG. 103

In the more advanced position the sole of the foot is held and the head rests on the knee. You will find this one of the most relaxing of all postures. If this position cannot be attained without discomfort, revert to the ankle. Remember that the elbows always bend outward during the stretch.

Hold for 10.

FIG. 104

When Fig. 103 can be accomplished with ease, substitute this extreme posture, holding the toes and bringing the elbows down toward the floor.

Hold for 10.

Following the 3 stretches with the left leg, slowly straighten to the upright position and relax for a few moments.

Stretch the right leg out, bring the left leg in; place the sole high against the right thigh.

Now perform the identical 3 stretching movements, once each, with the right leg.

Slowly straighten up, stretch the left leg out and relax.

The movements may be easier for you on one side than the other. If so, the Alternate Leg Stretch, along with Rishi's Exercise which we learned earlier, will help to balance the sides. If you concentrate on the movements, you will feel how each area of the leg (and back) is stretched through the 3 positions.

Summary: we do this exercise 3 times with each leg as follows: once to the calf, once to the ankle, once to your most extreme position. If you cannot hold the feet or toes, then you do 2 to the ankles. If you cannot hold the ankles, then you simply do 3 to the calves. Hold each stretch for 10.

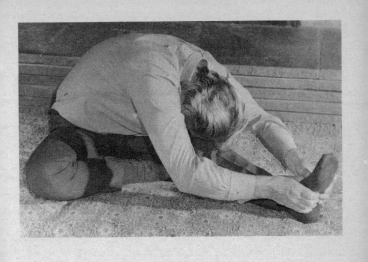

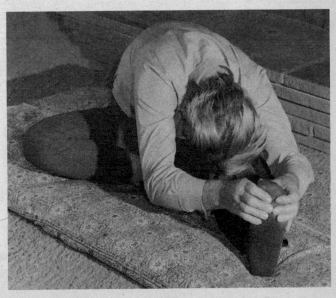

KNEE AND THIGH STRETCH
(30 seconds)

In this exercise we remove tension in the knees and thighs by bending the legs outward. It feels good to stretch the legs in a way seldom done during the course of our usual activities.

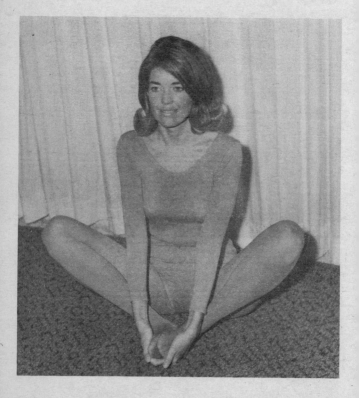

FIG. 105

Sit erect. Place the soles of your feet together and draw them in toward you as far as possible. Clasp your hands around your feet.

Pull up on your feet and bring your knees down as far as possible. Make sure to sit erect, don't slump.

Hold your extreme position for 10.

Relax the legs and bring the knees back to the original position of Fig. 105.

Repeat once.

Your extreme position is simply a question of structure. It doesn't matter how far down your knees actually go; a few inches are sufficient to benefit you. Just hold your extreme position motionless for 10 and you will stretch away the tension as well as firm the thighs and loosen the knees.

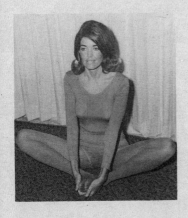

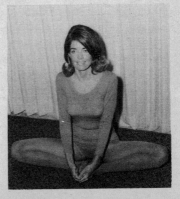

BACKWARD BEND
(1 minute)

In a previous routine we had occasion to remark how the exercise of the eyes was seriously neglected. We can state that the same is true of the feet. People do all kinds of exercises for many parts of their bodies, but seldom are the feet given the special attention they should have to help prevent the various troubles that do occur.

It is a generally known (and felt) fact that the shoes worn for most types of work, as well as for most social occasions, are harmful to the feet. Since many people wear shoes as much as twelve or more hours daily, it is small wonder that there is so much stiffness and general discomfort of the feet and toes and weakness in the ankles. Certain footwear can minimize these difficulties and you might want to look into this. I would urge that when you are at home you wear shoes—any kind of shoes—as little as possible; they're deadly. At any rate, here is an exercise designed so that you can carefully place extra weight on your feet and, in so doing, strengthen them. The "heels" position will also eliminate stiffness and tension. Although I teach this exercise primarily for the feet, the back and chest are also brought into play in a valuable manner.

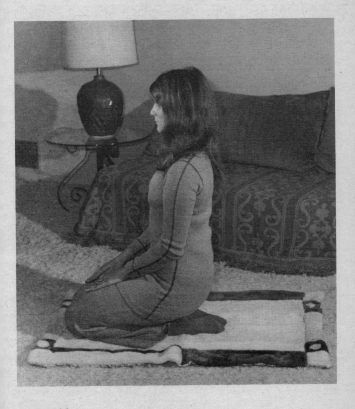

FIG. 108

Sit as illustrated with your full weight on your heels. Knees remain together throughout the exercise.

FIG. 109

Very slowly and cautiously inch your way a short distance backward with your hands. Do not go more than a short distance and do not "lunge" backward.

Now check your position to be sure that your arms are parallel with your sides and that all fingers are together and pointing directly behind you.

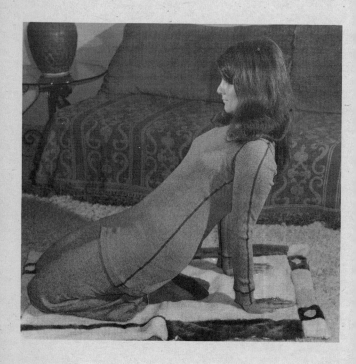

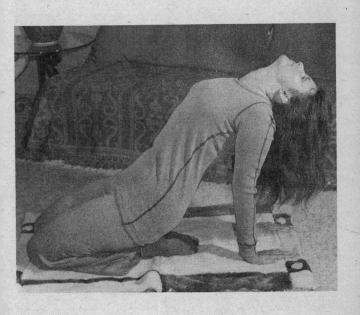

FIG. 110

Arch your back inward and lower your head as far back as possible. Remain seated on your heels (sometimes there is a tendency to raise the buttocks from the heels).

Hold without movement for 10.

FIG. 111

Raise your head and relax your trunk.

Now *very slowly* inch backward as far as you can go without strain. The arms must remain parallel to the sides and the fingers continue to point directly behind you.

Again, arch your back and lower your head.

Hold for 10.

Relax the trunk and head and *very slowly* inch your way forward to the original position of Fig. 108. Do not lunge forward.

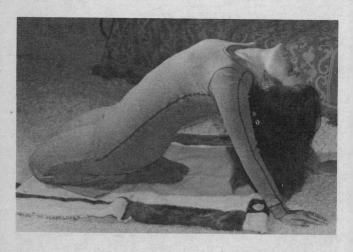

FIG. 112

Change the position of your feet so that the toes are on the floor as illustrated.

Very slowly and cautiously put as much weight as possible on your heels.

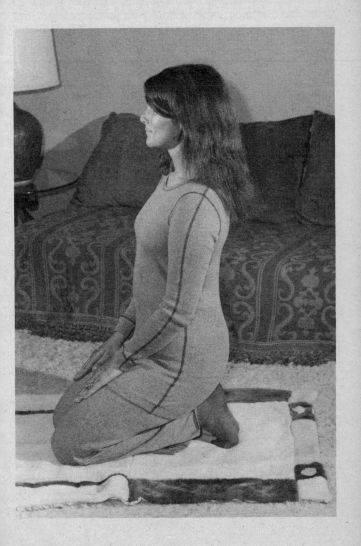

FIG. 113

A closeup view of the position.

In my classes it is not uncommon to hear numerous gasps and a number of shrieks of pain as students attempt this position and the subsequent position of Fig. 114 for the first time. This is because they disregard my warning of "slowly and cautiously" and just plop down onto their heels. The feet and ankles may have become seriously weak and stiff and they cannot immediately support the full weight of this position. The whole point of this exercise is to work out this stiffness and to strengthen the feet through applying the extra weight; but this may have to be done little by little, and for only a few moments at a time. So lower yourself slowly onto your heels (supported by your hands or fingertips that are resting on the floor) and "test" the situation. If it's painful, remain on your heels for just a few seconds with as much weight as is comfortable. Then raise yourself and try once or twice more. That's sufficient for the day. If you have the patience to practice this way, you'll be surprised at how quickly you rebuild the necessary strength in your feet and toes to support more and more of your weight. Within a few days, or possibly weeks, you should be able to sit on your heels with your full weight, and you will know that you have done yourself an important service. Stiffness and weakness in the feet can be a sure sign of trouble later on, so take whatever time is necessary now to work through these conditions. With few exceptions, mostly seriously overweight individuals, I have never taught this exercise to anyone who, with correct practice, has not mastered it within two months.

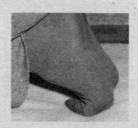

FIG. 114

When you feel comfortable in Fig. 112 very slowly and cautiously inch your way backward as before (although now it's more difficult because your trunk is considerably higher). Use your fingertips to go back only a few inches in the beginning and later on gradually increase the distance.

Now rest your palms on the floor. Make sure that your arms, hands, and fingers are exactly as illustrated.

Arch your spine and lower your head as before.

At first, hold your extreme position, whatever it may be, for 10. Gradually attempt to increase the count to 20. But come out of it at any point that discomfort is experienced.

Slowly lower your trunk, raise your head, and very slowly and cautiously inch your way forward with your hands and fingertips. Do not lunge forward.

Swing your legs around and extend them in front of you. Relax. If there is any discomfort in your feet massage them or manipulate the toes with your hands.

Summary:

Each time you do this exercise you perform the following positions:

Tops of the feet rest on floor—moderate distance back—hold 10

Tops of the feet rest on floor—move to extreme position—hold 10

Toes rest on floor—your extreme position (even if it is only sitting lightly on the heels without moving backward)—hold 10–20 (or less if necessary)

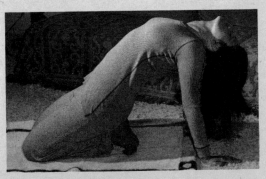

SHOULDER STAND
(3 minutes)

One of the most invaluably heathful things that you can do for yourself at the end of each workday is to invert your body. The profound regenerative effect of this simple maneuver on the entire organism is truly remarkable. We utilize several different techniques to accomplish this inversion in our various Yoga routines, and here it is the Shoulder Stand that we apply. Many Yoga students have come to regard the Shoulder Stand as one thinks about an old friend: enjoyable, reliable, always ready to help. Those people who glance at this posture in books, or happen to see it demonstrated in the media, and who dismiss it as irrelevant to their own needs do a great disservice to themselves. There is no living being who, unless he is suffering from some severe condition that would indicate otherwise, does not stand to benefit inestimably from taking a few minutes to reverse the flow of the blood. Technically, the Shoulder Stand does not actually reverse the circulation, but it feels as if this is happening. When we invert the body we feel pressure relieved in the legs, groin, and abdomen, and we feel the blood supply increased in the heart, chest, thyroid, and head. Most of our working positions offer no relief from the predominately downward flow of the blood. Remember that your heart is always pumping *against* gravity to bring the blood into the areas of the organism situated above it. With the Shoulder Stand we assist the heart in this function. One of the most interesting side effects of the Shoulder Stand is its ability to help regulate and redistribute weight. The thyroid gland is an important factor in weight control, and the increased supply of blood that is brought directly into the thyroid gland (because of the way the head is held at a right angle to the body) often provides the natural stimulation needed for a sluggish thyroid. There are other benefits: pressure is temporarily relieved in the arteries and veins of the legs, resulting in their relaxation (many workers will prop their legs up on a chair or desk for a few minutes during the day, intuitively seeking this type of relaxation); organs and glands of the viscera that may be prolapsed can often be returned to their correct positions, at least temporarily; it has had a salutary effect in uterine and prostate gland conditions; while the flow of the blood into the head is not as extreme as in the Headstand, it is still sufficient to aid in revitalizing the brain. You can now realize, at least intellectually, the value of serious effort to master the Shoulder Stand.

Keep a watch or clock nearby where you can see it. We need to time the extreme position.

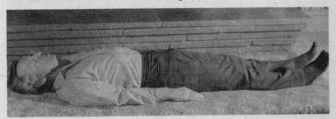

FIG. 115

From the seated position of the Backward Bend (your legs are extended in front of you) very slowly lower your back to the floor. Lie flat on your back with your arms at your sides and allow your body to go completely limp for a few moments. Nothing is held tensed.

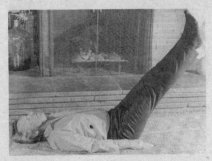

FIG. 116

Brace your palms firmly against the floor; tense your abdominal and leg muscles and slowly raise your legs with the knees straight.

FIG. 117

Swing your legs back over your head with sufficient momentum to allow your hips to leave the floor. Now bring your hands against your hips and support your trunk. If you have difficulty getting your hips off the floor, attempt to swing your legs back with increased momentum. In the beginning stages a few raisings and lowerings of the legs may be required to gain the necessary momentum for the swing of the legs over your head.

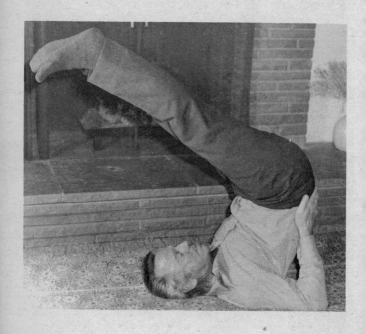

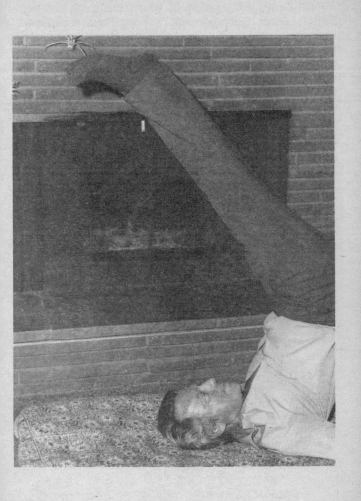

FIG. 118
Very slowly begin to straighten the legs and trunk. Go only as far as is comfortable. Any angle of inversion is adequate at first.

151

FIG. 119

The completed position in which the trunk and legs form a perfect right angle with the head; the chin is pressed against the chest. The body need not be held rigid; it is straight but relaxed. Hold whatever extreme position you attain comfortably for 1 to 2 minutes. Focus your full attention on your breathing and attempt to breathe slowly and rhythmically (keep your attention on your breathing; don't allow the mind to wander).

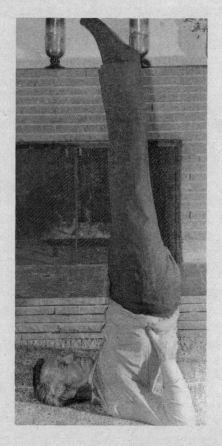

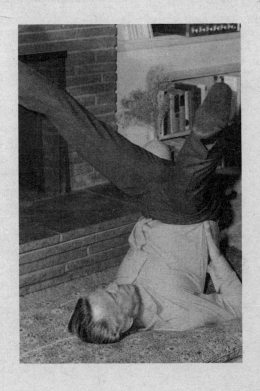

FIG. 120

Following the 1 to 2 minute hold, very slowly perform this "split" with the legs.

Hold for 10.

FIG. 121

Holding the legs apart, very slowly twist the trunk as far as possible to the left. It is the trunk that twists, the legs maintain their "split" position.

Hold for 10.

Now very slowly revolve the trunk to the extreme right. Again, the trunk is doing the twisting, not the legs.

Hold for 10.

Continue to hold the "split" and slowly return the trunk to the frontward position of Fig. 120.

Bring the legs together so that you are back in the position of Fig. 119 or Fig. 118.

It is absolutely essential to come out of the Shoulder Stand as smoothly and gracefully as possible so follow these directions carefully.

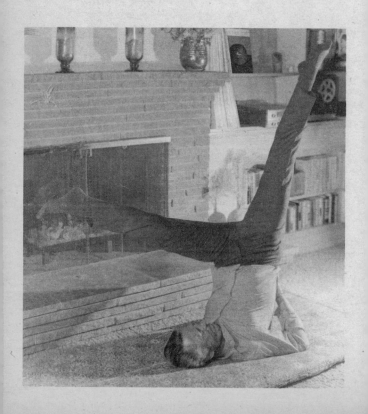

FIG. 122

Very slowly lower your knees as far as possible toward your head.

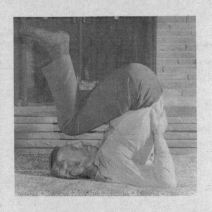

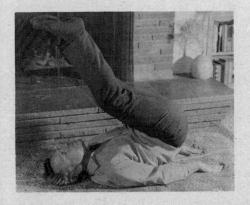

FIG. 123

Place your palms firmly against the floor. With as much control as possible, very slowly and smoothly begin to roll the trunk forward. As you do this, arch your neck. This arching will enable the back of your head to remain on the floor. We do not want the head to come up as we roll forward.

FIG. 124

When your hips touch the floor, extend your legs straight upward.

FIG. 125

Very slowly lower your legs to the floor with your knees straight. (This is an excellent movement for toning the muscles of the abdomen and legs; the slower you can lower the legs, the better.)

When the legs are once again resting on the floor, allow your body to go completely limp. Close your eyes.

If, due to a serious overweight problem or perhaps an acute weakness of certain muscles, you are unable to raise your hips from the floor in Fig. 117, I would advise you to use the wall as an aid. Lie parallel to and against the wall. Then swing your legs around, brace your feet against the wall, and simply "walk up" as far as you can. This may seem awkward at first, but you'll soon get the knack of it, and since any angle of inversion will be beneficial you should experiment and make whatever effort is necessary. This technique of using the wall may soon impart sufficient facility for you to perform the exercise without its aid.

In Figs. 118 and 119 remember to hold the body relaxed. If you are rigid and tense you will tire quickly. You needn't be in a hurry to attain Fig. 119. It will evolve naturally from Fig. 118 with a little practice. In the beginning your breathing may tend to be shallow and erratic, so concentrate on making it deep and rhythmic. You can glance at your watch or clock to time yourself. The 1 to 2 minute hold will go very quickly, especially if you are concentrating fully on your breathing. After approximately 2 weeks of practice the length of the hold in the extreme position can be increased. Whenever you are in the proper mood, and your time permits, you can hold the position for 3 to 5 minutes.

If, due to the pressure, you experience any discomfort in your neck or cervical vertebrae during the hold, you can place a folded towel underneath this area of your neck before you begin the exercise.

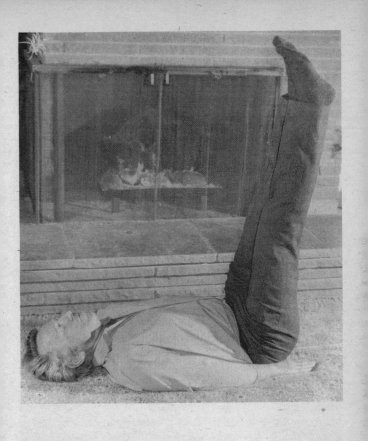

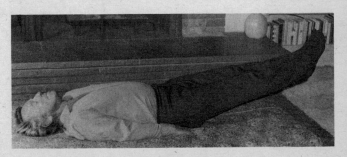

BREATHING
(1 minute)

We will conclude this 10 minute routine with approximately 1 minute of breathing for revitalization.

FIG. 126
Having completed the Shoulder Stand and rested briefly in this position, we will now take a very deep Complete Breath (remaining in the lying position). You will recall that the Complete Breath consists of a deep exhalation through the nose followed by a very deep inhalation performed slowly enough so that there is time for the abdomen to be distended and then the chest area expanded. When the chest is expanded to its fullest, hold the breath in your lungs. The raising of the shoulders will not be executed in this lying position. Keep your eyes closed.

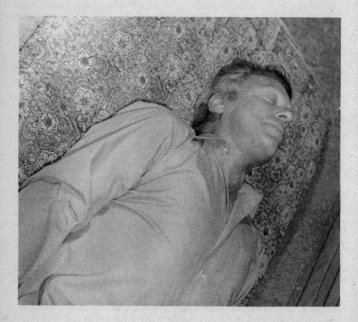

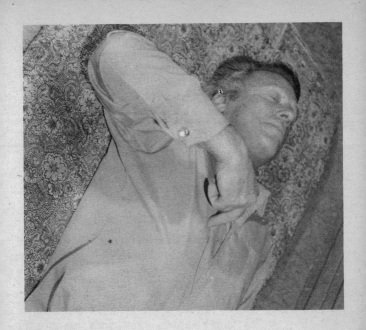

FIG. 127

Retaining the air deep in your lungs, tap the entire chest vigorously with the middle finger of your right hand. The technique is similar to the way in which a physician taps your chest when listening to your lungs—hammerlike and rhythmic. This forceful tapping will provide natural stimulation. Tap for as long as you can retain your breath comfortably (probably 15–30 seconds), and during this time begin by tapping in the highest area of the chest— the clavicle—and tap across in rows, backward and forward, moving down slightly each time until you are in the area of the lower lungs. Then exhale slowly and deeply, place your hand back down at your side and relax for as long as you wish.

Once is sufficient.

From this 10 minute "Returning Home" routine you will discover you gain a sort of "second wind"—renewed vitality and restoration of emotional equilibrium. These should now prevail for the remainder of your evening.

DINNER

(See the section on "Nutrition")

BEFORE RETIRING
(a 10 minute routine)

In the beginning pages of this book we noted that *sleep* was the most important state for regeneration of the life-force, the *prana* of the organism. We must have sufficient sleep or everything suffers—our minds, emotional stability, and efficiency. How many hours constitute "sufficient" sleep? Only you know. But whatever the number is you must make absolutely certain that you get it. The quickest way to jeopardize your health is consistently failing to sleep, in a restful manner, the necessary number of hours.

We have all experienced different types of sleep: fitful and troubled, exhausted, light, deep; possibly you have observed that it is the *deep* state, devoid of dreams, that provides the greatest regeneration and from which you awaken the most refreshed. One hour of truly deep sleep is worth eight of fitful tossing and turning. Of course, we all know that it is difficult to experience a deep, trouble-free sleep, or often any sleep at all, if the mind is disturbed with worry or excitement or the body is in pain through illness, indigestion, and so forth. But I would also point out that deep, restful sleep eludes that organism that is tense or exhausted. Exhaustion usually does not result in deep sleep but rather in fitful sleep. And tension that continually accumulates in key areas can inhibit a restful sleep without our conscious knowledge. You may awaken exhausted after a full night's sleep and not be aware that various types of tension have prevented your organism from gaining the necessary regeneration.

So, having established both the value of a restful sleep and the fact that certain conditions can inhibit it, we realize the efficacy of taking a few minutes to help eliminate these conditions, specifically, to remove physical tensions and quiet the mind and emotions. The Cobra, Alternate Nostril Breathing and Deep Relaxation exercises that follow will help provide this quietude. But in addition to these there are three good nighttime exercises (Lion, Scalp and Chin) that we can do in about three minutes to promote the health and appearance of areas that are seldom exercised. These latter three do not directly relate to our "restful sleep" objective (although they do remove certain tensions) and can be considered optional, to be performed, if you're going to do them, prior to the "quieting" exercises.

This routine should be performed as the last thing you do before retiring.

LION
(1 minute, 45 seconds)

Through the years this facial exercise has given all concerned a good many laughs. The various incidents that students have related to me (having to do mostly with the reactions of those who have come upon them unexpectedly while they were performing the Lion) would provide material for an extremely humorous chapter. But I will leave this to your imagination. The casual observer, already convinced that such postures as the Lotus and Headstand establish incontrovertibly the madness of the Yogi, finds the Lion Posture to be the ultimate proof of his convictions. It would certainly seem that by sticking out his tongue and making such a fierce face, the Yogi wishes to display his utter contempt for the world at large and is not adverse to altering his appearance in a most unflattering way in the process. While it is true that some relief of hostilities may be experienced through the Lion, its primary objective is less psychological: it happens to be one of the most complete and effective facial exercises you can do. It relieves tension and acts as a powerful firming agent. With one movement the muscles of the face, eyes, chin, and neck are simultaneously brought into play and toned. In spite of the development of the most ingenious exercise machines and cosmetics, firming and muscle toning remain essentially *internal* matters. No machine or cosmetic is able to firm your muscles. Only you can do this through your own muscular movements. Indeed, this is the case with all muscles of the body (as we shall see presently with our "Firming and Strengthening" routine); those of the face and neck are no exceptions. To help prevent or retard sagging of the face and neck you must maintain the tone of the muscles that support the skin; there are no better movements for this than those of the Lion. True, you may feel a bit foolish at first, when you stick out your tongue, but everyone does. Very quickly the novelty wears off, and when you note the visible improvements in your skin tone within two to three weeks of practice, the Lion will assume real importance for you. Use your cosmetics, lotions, and gadgets as you wish; they all have some value. But remember that true tone results from your own movements and that a youthful complexion is contingent primarily on exercise and diet.

My experience has been that many men shy away from facial exercises. I have never understood the reasoning behind this. Tension and sagging in the face, chin, and neck is certainly as prevalent in men as in women, possibly more so. Exercising the neck and facial muscles is no less important than exercising any other set of muscles, and I would therefore urge our male readers not to neglect the Lion and Chin exercises.

FIG. 128

Sit on the soles of your feet, exactly as we did in the first part of the Backward Bend. (If this presents a problem, sit in the Half-Lotus or the simple cross-legged posture.) Rest your hands, palms downward, on your thighs or knees. Relax completely.

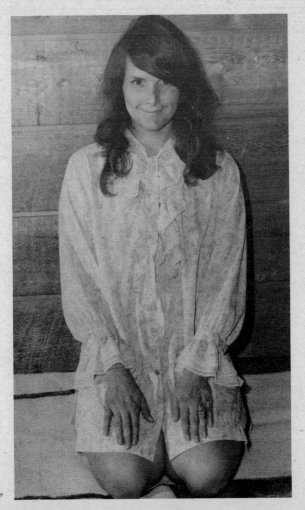

Move your trunk forward, open your eyes as wide as possible, tense the muscles throughout your body, spread your fingers wide and hold them this way, extend your tongue out and down as far as possible—as though you would touch your chin. Feel every muscle in the face and neck tighten. (Think ferociously, remember you're a lion. If you play it "chicken" and simply pop your tongue out an inch or so, you cannot tighten all the necessary muscles and you will not derive the benefits.)

Hold this tensed position for a count of 20. Do not allow any muscles to relax during this hold.

In very slow motion withdraw your tongue, relax all muscles, and settle back onto your heels. This slow withdrawal and settling back is done with a catlike movement.

Relax completely for a few seconds.

Perform 3 to 5 times.

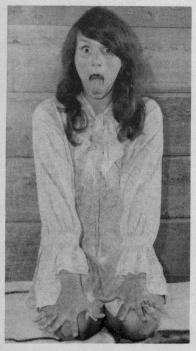
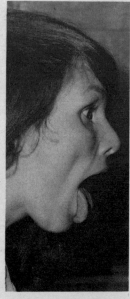

SCALP EXERCISE
(30 seconds)

Most women and many men are constantly concerned about the appearance of their hair; an incredible amount of time is devoted to washing, combing, brushing, setting, and the applying numerous tonics, colorings, dyes, and so forth. Yet the source of the health and beauty of the hair—the scalp—is almost always neglected. Other than shampooing most people do not think about giving special attention to the care of the scalp.

There are two things we can do for the scalp that will promote its health and simultaneously impart a natural luster to the hair: bring the blood into it and exercise it. Inverted postures such as the Shoulder Stand and Headstand as well as the Plough and Locust increase the blood supply into the head and nourish the follicles. Exercising the scalp will be accomplished by *moving* it. You will find that where baldness has occurred the scalp is tight, so we reason that keeping the scalp loose may prevent hair from falling out. Also, after this exercise we are about to do, your scalp will feel refreshed and stimulated. If we can speak about "tension" being present in the scalp, it seems to be removed through these movements.

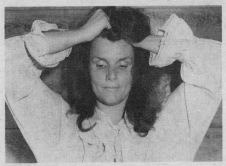

FIG. 130

With both hands, reach down into the roots of the front part of your scalp and take hold of as much hair as you can.

FIG. 131

Pull forward and backward very firmly so that your scalp moves. These are strong tugging movements, don't be too gentle. The hair should pull and the scalp feel pinched.

Do 15 of these forward-backward movements rhythmically and in continuous motion. There is no pause.

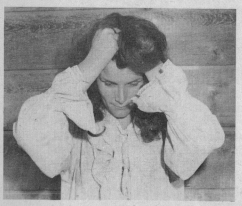

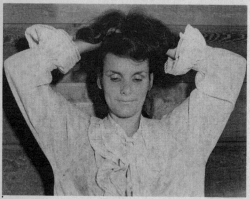

FIG. 132

Move your hands to the back part of the scalp and hold the hair partially at the sides and partially at the back of your head. Perform 15 of the same rhythmic forward-backward movements in continuous motion.

CHIN AND THROAT EXERCISE
(45 seconds)

FIG. 133

If comfortable, remain seated on your feet; otherwise, assume any seated position.

Allow your jaw to slacken so that your mouth is open slightly.

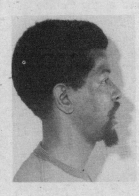

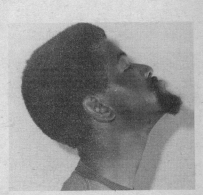

FIG. 134

In very slow motion, tilt your head backward, protrude your jaw and raise it as high as possible. Feel the skin in the chin and throat grow taut.

Hold for 5.

Slowly slacken the jaw and repeat the movements.

Perform 5 times. If you have a chin and/or throat problem you can perform 10 or more times.

COBRA
(2 minutes, 30 seconds)

It is probable that for a complete and immediate removal of tension throughout the spine and back, the Cobra is the most effective of all Yoga *asanas*. If you're troubled with your back during sleep, the Cobra is a "must." You may not realize how much tension you are harboring until you experience the relaxation induced by the Cobra.

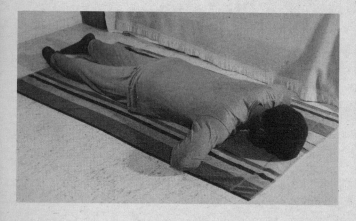

FIG. 135

Lie with your forehead resting on your mat.

Place your hands about 6 inches apart beneath your shoulders; all fingers are together and point directly toward the opposite hand. The position of the hands govern the movements so make sure you have it correct.

FIG. 136
In *the slowest motion possible;* repeat: *in the slowest motion possible,* arch your neck and raise only your head.

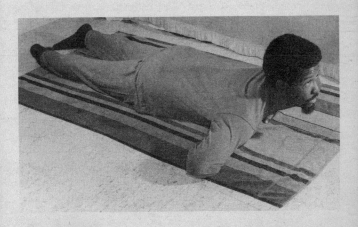

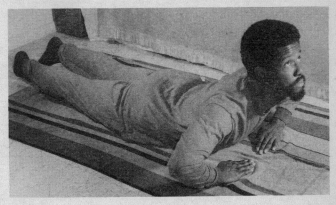

FIG. 137
Push against the floor with your palms and in very slow motion begin to raise the trunk. *Your spine must be curved* and your head back.

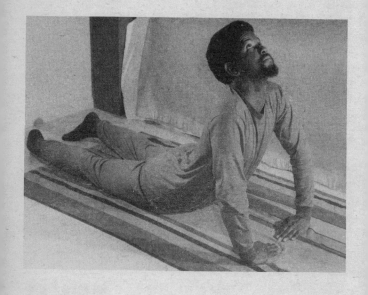

FIG. 138

Continue to raise your trunk with the spine curved. The motion is so slow that you can feel the pressure on each vertebra in turn. Concentrate on this transfer of pressure from one vertebra to the next. Head is back, eyes look upward.

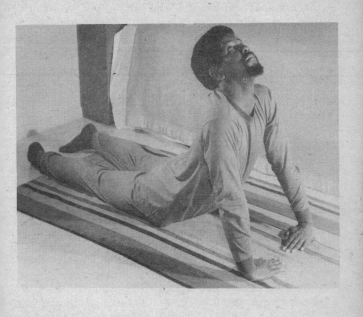

FIG. 139

The extreme position. Elbows are now straight but your spine is acutely curved, head back as far as possible, eyes look upward. Your legs must be relaxed (they have a tendency to tense). Pressure should be felt in the lowest lumbar vertebrae.

There is no hurry to accomplish this extreme position. Hold whatever position you have attained comfortably for a count of 20.

FIG: 140

From your extreme position bend your right elbow (the left remains straight) and very slowly twist your trunk to the left until you can see your left heel.

Hold for 10.

Slowly return to the frontward position of Fig. 139.

FIG. 141

Bend your left elbow (the right remains straight) and very slowly twist your trunk to the right until you can see your right heel.

Hold for 10.

Slowly return to the frontward position. Remember that here your trunk is once again raised as high as possible without strain. To come out of the posture simply reverse the movements: in the slowest motion possible, lower your trunk to the floor, making absolutely certain that the spine is continually arched every inch of the way. Again, concentrate fully on the pressure shifting from one vertebra to the next, from the lumbar all the way to the cervical. Do not allow the legs to stiffen and do not let gravity pull you down too fast. Bear in mind that it is the exaggerated slow motion that acts to remove tension and fatigue in this exercise.

When your forehead touches the mat, relax a few moment but keep the hands in their position beneath the shoulders.

Repeat the entire routine.

Upon completion, bring your arms back to your sides, rest your cheek on your mat, and allow your entire body to rest, completely limp.

At this point, having done the Cobra twice, you will feel so relaxed you will probably want to go right to sleep—but hold on; there are two more profound "quieting" exercises to do.

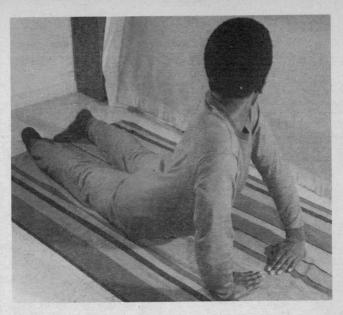

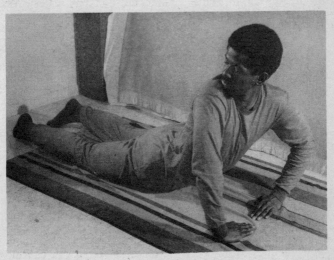

ALTERNATE NOSTRIL BREATHING
(3 minutes, 30 seconds)

One of the most startling concepts in the *Hatha* Yoga study comes to our attention in this breathing exercise: *the nostrils are not the same; the air that enters the right nostril fulfills a different function than that which is breathed through the left!*

Everywhere in the external world we see manifestations of the positive-negative principle: in the composition of the atom, in the cell, in the polarity of the earth, in the sun-moon relationship, in the existence of man-woman. In the inner, unseen worlds, those dimensions of existence we gradually come to perceive through our inner or "third" eye, the same positive-negative phenomenon obtains. And just as in the external world we know that a certain balance must always be maintained in the positive-negative ratio, so in our subtle or "astral" bodies a balance must be maintained in the constant interplay of positive-negative currents. We are affected adversely according to the degree of imbalance. There are metaphysicians who will diagnose many physical illnesses, as well as emotional or mental disturbances, as an "imbalance in the positive-negative forces."

The primary source of *prana* is in the air we breathe. The *prana* is broken into positive and negative elements as it enters the nostrils. The word *Hatha* is composed of two Sanskrit syllables: "ha" represents the sun, and "tha" represents the moon. Symbolically, Yogis have applied "ha" to the right or "sun" (warm) nostril, and "tha" to the left or "moon" (cool) nostril. The actual routes and functions of the prana as it travels through the channels of the subtle body require more esoteric discussion than this book is designed to provide (although I will treat the subject of the physiological aspects of the subtle body in a subsequent book). However, we can make very practical use of the above information regarding the positive-negative principle at this point where we are applying a number of techniques to induce a restful sleep. Here you can aid in the correction of imbalances that may exist in your emotional and mental bodies, conditions that have built up during the day and can prevent a sound sleep. *We will now make a very deliberate attempt to balance the positive-negative ratio by breathing slowly and rhythmically through the nostrils in an alternate manner.* Like the Cobra this exercise has the most immediate and profound quieting effect on the entire organism, including its mental and emotional aspects.

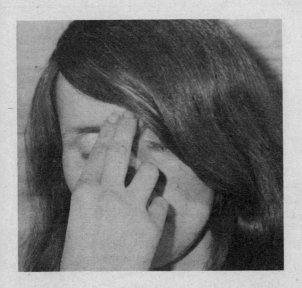

FIG. 142

The Half-Lotus or simple cross-legged posture is best for this exercise. You should not have to move your legs, and you must keep your spine erect for its duration, so find a suitable position.

Rest your left hand on your left thigh.

Study the illustration. Place the tip of your right thumb lightly against the right nostril, and the ring finger and little finger lightly against the left. The index and middle fingers are together and they rest lightly on the forehead (in the "third eye" area). Exhale deeply, slowly, and as quietly as possible through both nostrils.

FIG. 143

When the exhalation is completed, immediately close your right nostril by pressing the thumb against it. Slowly and quietly inhale a deep breath through the left nostril. This inhalation is done during a rhythmic count of 8.

FIG. 144

Keep the right nostril closed and now press the *left* closed so that both nostrils are closed. Retain the air for a rhythmic count of 4.

FIG. 145

Release the *right* nostril (the left remains closed) and exhale slowly, deeply, and quietly in a rhythmic count of 8.

When the air is completely exhaled do not pause but immediately begin the next inhalation through the *right* nostril (this is the same nostril through which you just finished exhaling). Inhale a deep, quiet breath in a count of 8. The left nostril remains closed.

Keep the left nostril closed and now press the *right* closed so that once again both are closed. Retain the air deep in your lungs for a rhythmic count of 4.

Release the *left* nostril (the right remains closed) and exhale deeply and quietly in a rhythmic count of 8.

Now you have returned to the original starting point. Each time you return to this starting point you have completed one round of Alternate Nostril Breathing.

Without pause keep the right nostril closed and begin a deep, quiet inhalation through the *left*.

Perform 5 complete rounds.

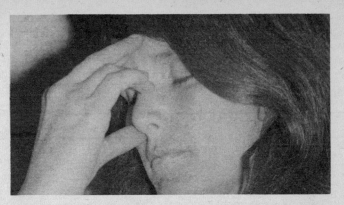

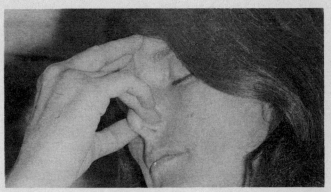

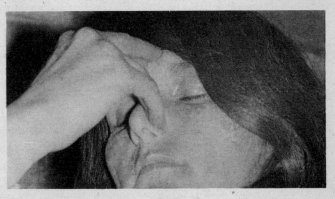

Summary:

inhale through left	count 8
hold breath; both nostrils are closed	count 4
exhale through right	count 8

without pause:

inhale through right	count 8
hold breath; both nostrils are closed	count 4
exhale through left	count 8

This completes one round. Then, without pause:

inhale through left	count 8
etc.	

Perform 5 rounds

Important: the counting for the breathing in groups of 8 and 4 is rhythmic and continuous. You never interrupt the counting; there are no pauses. Once you begin the count you keep it going in your mind steady and rhythmic like a metronome.

Don't allow the breath to "gush" or "hiss" in or out. Perform the inhalations and exhalations as quietly as possible. Think of the breathing being done more in the throat than the nostrils.

Once you have read through the instructions keep your eyes closed throughout the exercise and concentrate fully on your counting. Do not permit the mind to wander. At no time should this breathing become "automatic," that is, should the breathing continue but your attention be drawn elsewhere.

Keep your spine erect and your body relaxed throughout. If your legs tire, reverse them with the least possible movement.

DEEP RELAXATION
(1 minute)

We will now take one minute and conclude the routine with a very ancient Yoga technique. This should be done in bed with the lights out.

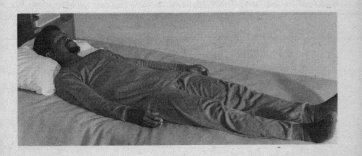

FIG. 146

Lie on your back, arms at your sides. Allow your body to go limp. Focus your full attention on your feet; if they are being held tensed in any way, relax them.

Next, become aware of your calves and knees; relax them completely. Now determine if all the muscles in your thighs are relaxed. Slowly draw your consciousness up into the lower abdomen, then the upper abdomen, then the chest. As you become aware of each of these areas in turn, make sure there are no muscular contractions. Now shift your attention to your fingers, then lower arms, upper arms, and shoulders. Again, "feel" the condition of each of these in turn and withdraw all support so that they are absolutely limp. Then determine if your neck is in the most comfortable position; if not, adjust it.

Finally, relax your jaw and face.

Become aware that your body is now in a state of deep relaxation. Exclude all thoughts and concentrate on your breathing; observe it for a short time exactly as we did the moment we awakened.

Shortly you should pass into a state of deep, restful sleep.

ADDITIONAL INFORMATION REGARDING
A RESTFUL SLEEP

Here are a number of suggestions that you will find helpful in promoting an undisturbed sleep:

Do not eat *anything* for two hours before retiring. This includes hot milk, tea, and other beverages and concoctions that supposedly help you sleep. You cannot sleep restfully if your digestion processes are at work. (Incidentally, sleeping pills are deadly. Take them only upon the urgent advice of your physician.)

Yogis recommend sleeping predominately on your right side. The theory is that pressure on the heart is eased. You can gain the awareness during sleep to know which side you are on. Try it.

Sleeping on a very firm surface and raising the head only slightly are also advised.

The Yogi positions himself during sleep so that his head is toward the north and his feet toward the south. This polarity is in harmony with that of the earth, and has a positive "magnetizing" effect. If you can do so, arrange your bed in this north-south position.

WEEKEND PRACTICE
(a 20–30 minute routine)

Now that you have had the opportunity to test the Yoga routines during the week and found that one or more of them really does work for you, you usually have the opportunity to undertake some additional practice over the weekend and significantly increase your benefits. For example, there are special Yoga exercises for firming and strengthening the entire body that also help regulate and control your weight on a permanent basis. The weekend is ideal for this routine which requires more time than we are able to devote, practically, during the week. The weekend is also good for learning and practicing the Headstand as well as perfecting various exercises that were included in our weekday routines.

Although some of my students have found it enjoyable to have other members of their families join them in this weekend practice I prefer that the same conditions of privacy prevail as during those routines that we did at home during the week. Get off by yourself for the necessary time and, in addition to this special weekend routine, include a few of those exercises that you found especially beneficial during the week. Spend a little additional time with these exercises; that is, perform several more repetitions than we did during the week and add some extra time to the extreme holds. An exercise such as the Shoulder Stand, for example, can be increased by as much as two minutes in your extreme position. The "Arising" and "Before Retiring" routines can be practiced at the usual times with increased repetitions and holding time in the various exercises if you wish.

HIP BEND
(1 minute, 30 seconds)

These movements will firm and help to reduce excess inches in your sides, hips, and waist.

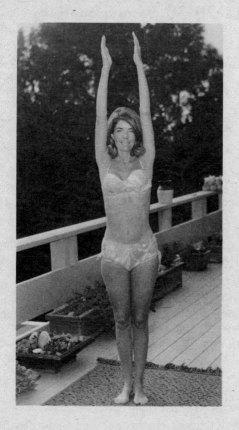

FIG. 147

Stand erect with your feet together. Slowly raise your arms overhead so that they are parallel. Palms face each other.

FIG. 148

Very slowly bend your trunk a moderate distance to the left side. Do not go as far as you can. Your arms must remain parallel.

Hold motionless for 10.

Very slowly straighten to the upright position and perform the same moderate bend to the right side.

Hold for 10.

Slowly straighten to the upright position.

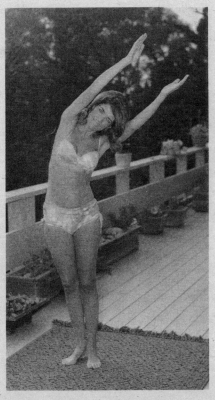

FIG. 149

Very slowly bend your trunk as far as possible to the left.

Your arms must remain parallel with each other; this is very important for firming. Relax your neck. Feel the tautness and firming action in your right side.
Hold for 10.
Slowly straighten to the upright position.
Perform the extreme bend to the right side.
Hold for 10.
Slowly straighten up and gracefully lower your arms to the sides. Rest for a few moments.
Repeat only the extreme bends to the right and left once.
Hold each for 10.
Upon completion lower yourself gracefully into a seated position and relax.

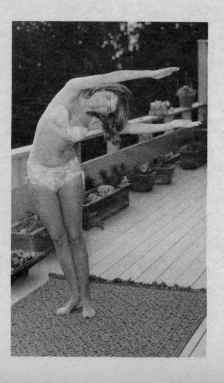

FULL TWIST
(1 minute, 30 seconds)

In an earlier routine we performed the Simple Spinal Twist while seated in a chair. This was to provide a quick, loosening movement and relief of tension in the spine. Now we will perform the Full Twist, a most powerful "corkscrew" series of movements, of which the Simple Twist is a modified position. Possibly you have observed that in this book we are involved in three basic spinal movements: *convex,* as in the Cobra and Bow, *concave* as in the Back Stretch and Plough, *spiral* or twisting as in Rishi's Exercise and now in the Full Twist. You may also have become aware that a great deal of the effectiveness in a number of the major Yoga exercises lies in the method by which they enable us to first assume a "lock" or "hold" and then stretch to any degree we desire *against* this lock. For example, in the Back Stretch and Alternate Leg Stretch the legs or feet are held and we stretch the back and spine concavely against this hold; in the Bow the feet are held as a lock and we manipulate the back and spine convexly against this lock. Here, in the Full Twist, the lock is a most ingenious one. You will note that in the position of Fig. 154 the full lock has been assumed, that is, the leg has locked the lumbar area of the spine, and the arm is holding this leg in place so that the dorsals and the cervical vertebrae can twist against the lock. There is an aspect of chiropractic in these manipulations against locks.

Of all the Yoga exercises the Full Twist has taken students the longest period of time to absorb. This is not because of the difficulty of the movements but rather because of their number; there are seven and you really have to think carefully about what you are doing in order to get the lock correctly set up. If you have ever seen me teach this exercise on television you may remember that I show many of the incorrect movements students make because they get themelves tied into some terrible knots and perform some strange twists. But here, with all of the details fully illustrated for you, you should have a minimum of trouble in learning the correct procedure.

Again, your efforts will be well rewarded because just as you have now experienced how the Cobra imparts the most wonderful and immediate relaxation to the entire back, so will you feel how the Full Twist results in an immediate replenishment of vitality. When the spine is loosened in this spiral fashion there seems to be an instantaneous release of trapped energy.

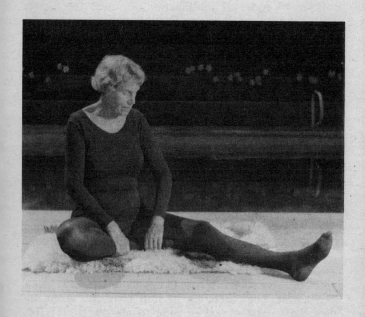

FIG. 150

You have assumed a seated position following the Hip Bend exercise. Now extend your legs straight outward.

Take hold of your right foot and bring the heel as far in as possible; the sole rests flat against your upper left thigh.

FIG. 151

Bring your left leg in so that you can take a firm hold on your left ankle with both hands.

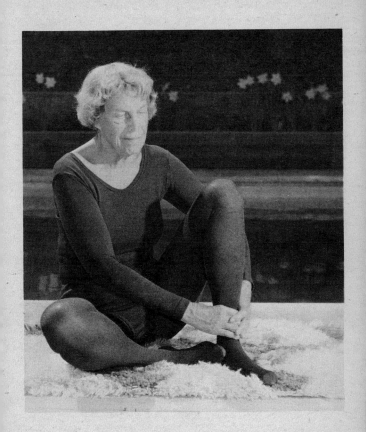

FIG. 152

Study the photograph. You now move your left foot over your right knee and place it firmly on the floor adjacent to your right knee. Look at the photograph again and make sure you have the position correct.

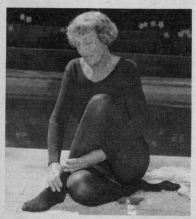

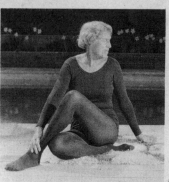

FIG. 153

We are still in the process of setting up the "lock." The right hand remains on the ankle but the *left* hand is placed firmly on the floor behind you. This is to provide support and balance for the next movement.

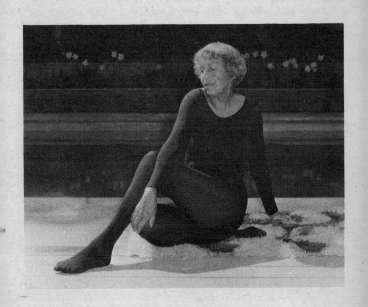

FIG. 154

This is the critical movement and completes the lock.

Remove your right hand from your ankle and slowly bring it *over* (not under) your left leg.

Take a firm hold on your right knee with your right hand. You will now feel how the lumbar area has been locked. If your big belly or arm prevents you from holding the knee as described, push your left foot farther out and away from your right knee. This should enable you to hold the right knee with ease. But subsequently work to bring the left foot in as close to the knee as you can because this position allows you to lock the spine quite high, and the higher, the better.

FIGS. 155A and 155B

Very slowly begin to turn your trunk and head as far to your *left* (note, *left* not right) as possible.

Simultaneously move your left hand from the floor to hold the right side of your waist.

Your head turns very far, as though you would rest it on your left shoulder. At first this position will feel tight, cramped, uncomfortable. But after just a few attempts the body adjusts to it easily. You can now feel this "spiral" or "corkscrew" position of the entire spine. This is also an excellent movement for helping to streamline your waist.

Hold without motion for 10.

Place your left palm down firmly on the floor and very slowly turn your trunk frontward so that you are once again in the position of Fig. 154.

Relax a few moments.

Repeat the twisting movement and hold for 10.

Return to the frontward position.

Take hold of your left foot with both hands and bring it back over the right knee to the position of Fig. 151.

Extend both legs outward.

Perform the identical movements on the opposite side by exchanging the words "right" and "left" in the above directions.

Do the twist twice to this right side and hold each for 10.

FIRMING, STRENGTHENING, AND DEVELOPING

In connection with the Lion exercise we stated that good muscle tone and firm, taut skin were primarily *internal* matters. Your muscles must retain tone to support your skin or it will become flabby and sag no matter what exercise machine, gadget, device, massager, or stimulator you use to push, pull, or manipulate. Only through your own movements can your muscles remain genuinely toned. Previously we were speaking about the face, but as we are about to see, this principle pertains to the entire body.

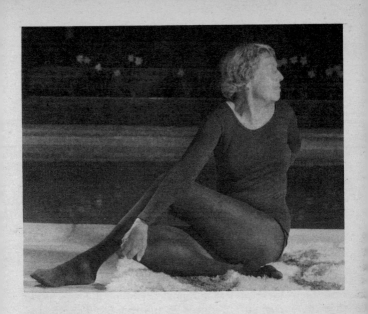

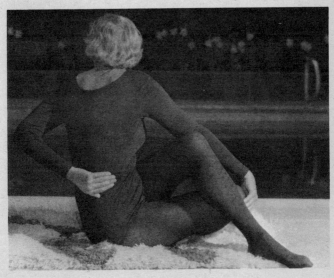

The Yoga movements that are designed to firm, strenghen, and develop are not strenuous and will not exceed your capacity regardless of your age or physical condition. Many people think of firming in terms of practices that are exhausting: innumerable repetitions; peddling, pushing, and pulling devices; weight lifting. In Yoga, however, a *passive* concept of muscular development obtains. It is not our intention to overtax the muscles, and we certainly have no wish to develop bulging biceps. Our plan is to make moderate demands, in accordance with your ability, upon each set of muscles throughout the body (without exhausting them) so that they retain their strength and resilience. If you are interested in additional development, you simply increase the holding time and number of repetitions. Sedentary workers have great need of these exercises since their muscles simply do not receive sufficient stress during the workweek.

It is also important to note that those of my students who have seriously practiced the following exercises to firm their muscles and eliminate flabbiness have found that excess weight is reduced in the process. Pounds and inches definitely seem to be more easily lost as well as redistributed when the body becomes firm. Further, these exercises will help to *keep the excess weight off*. You'll be pleasantly surprised at how quickly our firming routine (the following four exercises) produces the results you desire.

SIDE RAISE
(2 minutes)

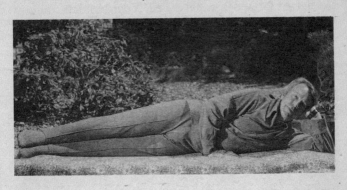

FIG. 156
From the sitting position of the Full Twist gracefully move into the illustrated lying position. You lie on your left side and support your head with your left hand; rest your right hand firmly against the floor.

FIG. 157
Push against the floor and very slowly raise your right leg as high as possible.

Hold for 10 as steady as possible.

Slowly lower the leg.

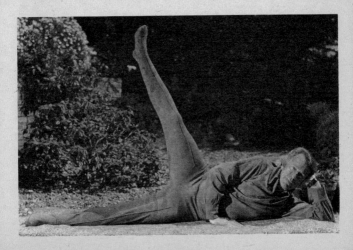

FIG. 158

Raise both legs a moderate distance from the floor. Do not go farther than illustrated. Your legs must remain together; they must come directly up from your side and must not sway frontward or backward.

Hold as steady as possible for 10.

Very slowly lower the legs to the floor.

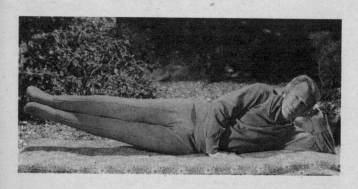

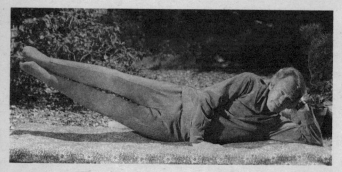

FIG. 159

Now raise both legs as high as possible; bring them directly up from the side and do not let them sway.

Hold for 10.

Very slowly lower the legs to the floor.

Relax a few moments but remain in the position of Fig. 156.

Repeat only the extreme position once.

Gracefully roll onto your right side and perform the identical movements: raise only the left leg first, then both legs a moderate distance, then both legs as high as possible twice. Hold each raise for 10.

Summary:

Left side	raise right leg only once	hold 10
	both legs; moderate raise once	hold 10
	both legs; extreme raise twice	hold 10 each
Right side	raise left leg only once	hold 10
	both legs; moderate raise once	hold 10
	both legs; extreme raise twice	hold 10 each

PLOUGH
(3 minutes)

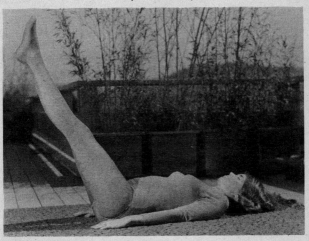

FIG. 160

From the Side Raise position gracefully roll onto your back. Rest your palms against the floor at your sides. Bring your legs together, push against the floor with your hands, and slowly and gracefully begin to raise your legs, knees straight.

FIG. 161

As in the Shoulder Stand, swing your legs back over your head *slowly, with control.* (If this slow movement is too difficult, you can swing them backward with more momentum.)

As slowly as possible begin to lower your feet to the floor. Go only an inch at a time so you can carefully "feel" your back and vertebrae stretching. Be absolutely certain to stop completely at that point where you begin to experience the slightest strain. The object in the initial days of practice is not to make the feet touch the floor but rather to slowly work out the areas of the back that are stiff and those vertebrae that are inflexible. The only way to do this permanently is to stop the downward movement of the legs at exactly the point where you begin to experience difficulty and hold your legs motionless at this point.

Hold whatever extreme position of the legs is comfortable for 20.

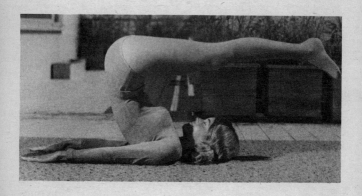

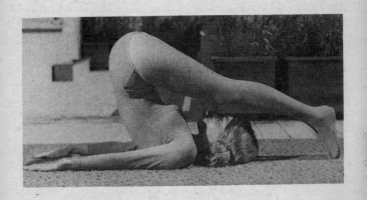

FIG. 162

As you gain the necessary flexibility your feet will touch the floor. There is no trick to this and it should never be done through sheer effort or momentum. It will happen naturally, and we are prepared to take several weeks or even months to accomplish this position.

Hold for 20.

Important: note that the feet are positioned relatively close to the head. The legs are not extended as far as possible behind you. In lowering the legs we make a deliberate attempt to aim the feet close in toward the head in order to place the pressure on the lower back, the lumbar vertebrae. Your knees must not bend. (Compare the position of the feet here with that of the *second* position in Fig. 168.

As with the Shoulder Stand it is important to come out of whatever extreme position you have held with grace and control. So follow these directions carefully:

197

FIG. 163
Bend your knees and begin to roll forward slowly.

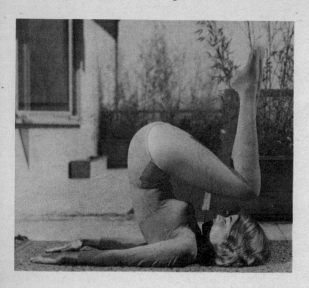

FIGS. 164 and 165

Brace your palms firmly against the floor and arch your neck. This will enable you to keep your head on the floor. Remember, we do not want the head to come up from the floor in this forward roll. When your hips touch the floor, extend your legs straight outward and slowly lower them to the floor.

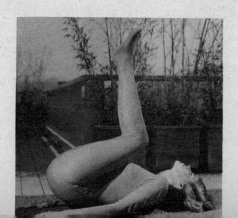

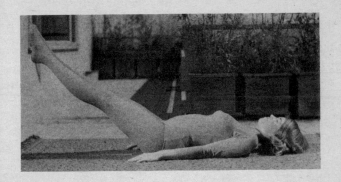

FIG. 166

Without pause, and as slowly as possible, begin to sit up with your arms extended. This is an excellent movement for toning the abdominal muscles; however, if it is too difficult keep your hands on the floor and give yourself a slight push upward until you can continue to raise your trunk without support—then extend your arms outward as illustrated.

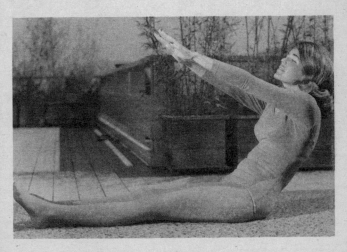

FIG. 167

When you have reached the upright sitting position, continue to stretch forward and take hold of the furthermost area of your legs you can reach (calves, ankles, feet) and perform one Back Stretch movement with your elbows bent.

Hold for 10.

Very slowly lie back down without the use of your hands (also for toning the abdomen).

Relax.

Repeat the entire routine once.

The following two additional positions cannot be performed until your feet have touched the floor comfortably, so do not attempt them unless you have accomplished Fig. 162.

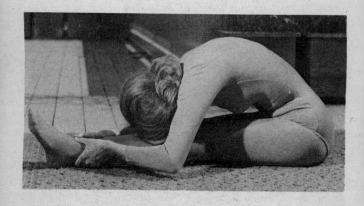

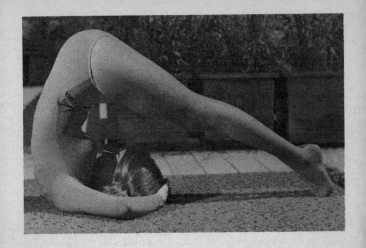

FIG. 168

After you have held the position of Fig. 162 for 20, slowly and gracefully bring your arms up from your sides and clasp your hands on the top of your head.

You will now be able to slowly move your toes a few inches farther back. If you do this very slowly and "feel" what is happening, you will sense that the pressure is being shifted from the lumbar to the middle area of your spine. Knees must be kept straight. Your breathing will be cramped at first but, as with the Shoulder Stand, the lungs will adjust after a few attempts.

Hold this *second* position of the Plough for 20.

FIG. 169

This peculiar looking position is actually one of the most comfortable of all Yoga postures! Of course, nobody believes this until he has tried it; once mastered it affords the most wonderful stretch for the entire back and spine with absolutely no effort.

Following your hold of 20 in the second position, lower your knees to the inside of your bent elbows. Go only an inch or two in the beginning and gradually you may be able to touch the knees to the floor. Now you will feel the transfer of the pressure again, this time from the middle to the upper (cervical) vertebrae. As in the second position breathing will be cramped during initial attempts; concentrate on breathing very slowly and rhythmically.

Hold this *third* Plough position for 20.

Come out of the position by rolling forward slowly. As you do this bring your arms back down to your sides gracefully and then simply follow the instructions already given in Figs. 163 thru 167.

Summary:

Your extreme position of the first position—hold 20
When you can:

    the second position   —hold 20
    the third position   —hold 20
The Back Stretch   —hold 10

Perform the entire routine (which includes whatever you can do of the Plough plus the Back Stretch) twice.

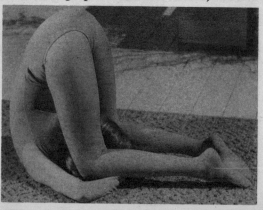

BACK PUSH-UP
(1 minute)

FIG. 170

You are lying on your back, having completed the Plough. Assume the position illustrated. Fingers rest on the floor pointing behind you and heels are drawn in as far as possible; knees and feet are together.

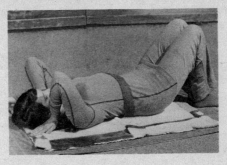

FIG. 171

Push your fingers and feet against the floor and raise your body as high as possible. Knees must remain together.

Hold as steady as possible for 10.

Slowly lower the body to the floor.

Repeat twice so that you do 3 in all.

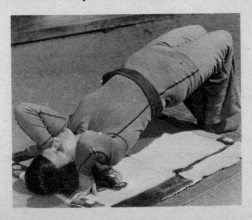

FIG. 172

An advanced position that must be executed cautiously. Push your fingers and feet against the floor and as you begin to raise your body, carefully arch your neck so that

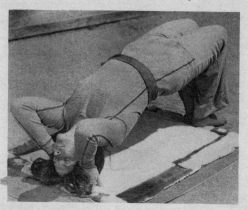

the top of your head rests on the floor. Raise as high as possible with knees together.

Hold as steady as you can for 10.

Slowly lower your body and cautiously move your head back to the original position while you are lowering.

When you once again rest on the floor, extend your legs outward and bring your arms back to your sides.

Relax.

The advanced position is done only once.

LOCUST
(2 minutes)

FIG. 173

Roll over gracefully so that your chin rests on your mat. Make fists of your hands and rest them firmly on the floor, thumbs down, next to your sides.

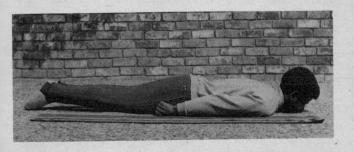

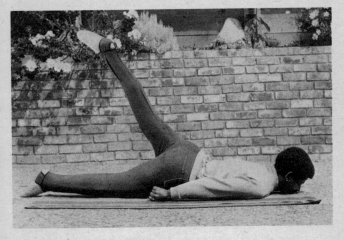

FIG. 174

Push your fists against the floor and very slowly raise your left leg as high as possible. Keep the knee straight.

Hold for 10.

Slowly lower the leg to the floor.

Perform the same movements with the right leg.

The above movements must be done very slowly to be effective in firming the lower abdomen, thighs, and legs.

FIG. 175

Take a breath and retain it.

Push down with your fists and raise both legs a moderate distance. Your chin remains on the floor and your legs are close together.

Do not go farther than illustrated.

Hold the raise and retain the breath for 10.

Slowly, with control, lower the legs to the floor.

Exhale. (You exhale only *after* the legs have touched the floor.) Relax a few moments; keep the chin on the mat.

FIG. 176

Take another breath (slowly) and retain it.

Now raise both legs as high as possible. The effort is what is important here, not how high you are able to raise. Your legs must be close together, knees straight, and your chin remains on the mat. (This is also an excellent strengthening and firming movement for the arms.)

Hold as steady as possible for 7. (Note: 7, not 10.)

Very slowly lower your legs to the floor.

Exhale slowly only after the legs have touched the floor. Control the exhalation, don't let the breath "gush" out.

Relax a few moments and get your "second wind."

Repeat the extreme position only twice, so that you do 3 of them in all. Hold each extreme raise for 7.

After completing the final repetition, turn your head so that your cheek rests on your mat and relax deeply for a minute or so.

This is not an easy exercise. It brings into play muscles of the lower abdomen that you very seldom exercise and, for this reason alone, is very valuable. It is simply a question of repeated attempts that will strengthen the necessary muscles and enable you gradually to raise the legs higher. Some people do a good raise the first time, but only a few inches is perfectly adequate. You may have seen us instruct Johnny Carson in this exercise on his show. He did a very respectable Locust—high collar shirt and tie included.

This series of movements requires the most muscular effort of all our Yoga exercises. The extreme position resembles the locust (or grasshopper) whose rear extremities are raised.

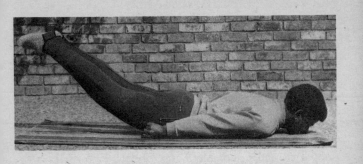

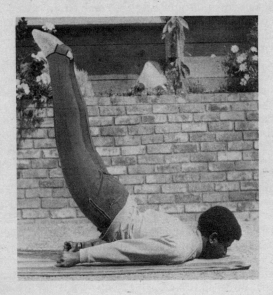

Summary:

Left leg once	hold 10
Right leg once	hold 10
Both legs (moderate raise with breath retained) once	hold 10
Both legs (extreme raise with breath retained) 3 times	hold 7 each

HEADSTAND
(3–5 minutes)

Right from the beginning I want to encourage you to try this posture; I have had a great deal of success in teaching students the Headstand. I attribute this success to emphasizing from the onset that we make no attempt to spring into a full Headstand like an accomplished acrobat; rather, we proceed with extreme caution to invert the body very gradually in a series of stages, feeling fully supported and in complete control each step of the way. I further stress that attaining the complete inversion need not necessarily be our objective because many important benefits are derived from even the most modified positions. Understanding this, students in our elementary classes who, prior to attending, had decided that they will absolutely never be able to do the Headstand are induced to at least try it—and are usually pleasantly surprised to find their efforts meeting with success.

Granted, some patient practice must be invested in this exercise. Is it worth it? Well, in addition to developing an acute sense of balance and imparting many benefits similar to those described under the "Shoulder Stand," the Headstand brings the blood *directly* into the head. Nothing else can so quickly refresh the brain and aid in clarity of the mind; you feel remarkably invigorated after a short period of time in this inverted position. The Headstand has brought about improvements in vision, hearing, and breathing; it also nourishes the complexion and scalp. Since this book is not primarily of an esoteric nature, I will mention the following only in passing: in addition to deriving important physical benefits (not all of which have been stated above), Yogis perform the Headstand to help stimulate brain power that lies dormant. For many centuries Yogis have maintained that most humans utilize only a fraction of what is a great untapped potential of brain power. The Headstand is one of the *asanas* that is designed to give us access to this potential. I have stated that it is my intention to discuss the esoteric aspect of the various *asanas* in a subsequent book.

Now that you know some theory regarding the Headstand, let us try it. It is the practice, not the theory, that is real—and this is always the truth of *Hatha* Yoga: you *do,* not talk; you *experience,* not theorize.

FIG. 177

From the completed position of the Locust, raise your trunk by bracing your hands against the floor and slowly settle back onto your heels. Have a small pillow nearby before you begin the entire Weekend routine and, at this point, place it as illustrated. The pillow serves to relieve pressure on the head and neck; eventually you may find that you don't need it, but it's a good idea to use it in the beginning stages. Also, position a clock or watch where you will be able to see it with your head down.

Extend your arms and interlace your fingers.

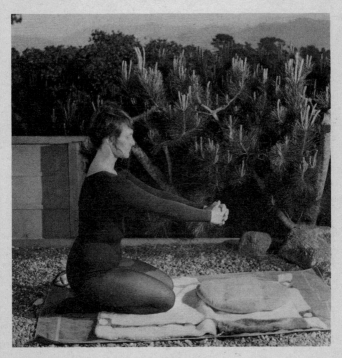

FIG. 178

Very slowly bend forward and place your hands on the mat. Rest your toes on the floor.

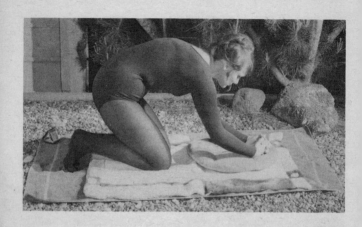

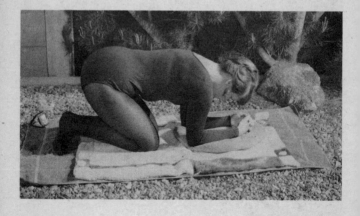

FIG. 179

Lower your elbows and forearms so that they form a triangle.

FIG. 180
Lower your head so that the top rests on the floor and the back is cradled firmly against your clasped hands. (Note: the back of the head does not rest on *top* of the hands but *against* them.)

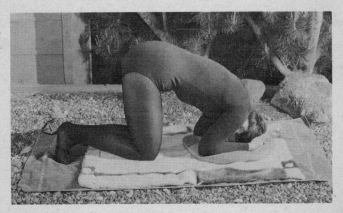

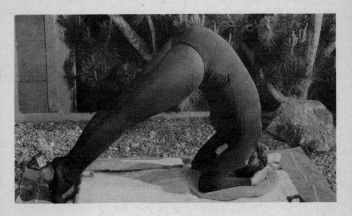

FIG. 181
Push down with your toes and forearms and raise your body into this arch.

Remain here a few moments until you feel secure in the position.

FIG. 182

Now very slowly lower your knees to about chest level.

This is as far as you should go the first few times. You will derive many benefits from this position, and you should not attempt the next positions until you feel absolutely secure and comfortable here.

Hold 30 seconds.

FIG. 183

To come out of the posture, lower your knees to the floor.

Next, move the legs back. Rest the tops of your feet on your mat. Remain with your head down, relaxing your muscles for approximately 30 seconds.

Slowly raise your head and come into a seated posture.

When you feel absolutely secure in Fig. 182, you should attempt the "Modified" Headstand.

FIG. 184

Push off the floor lightly with your toes and move your trunk forward. Attempt to transfer your weight so that it is evenly distributed between your head and forearms. This is a delicate maneuver; don't go lurching upward or you will probably tumble forward. You must keep your knees bent as far as possible and have them in toward your chest. Make no attempt to straighten your legs upward until this position is completely mastered or you will never really learn the Headstand.

If your feet fall back to the floor relax a few moments and try again. Three or four attempts are sufficient for any of the Headstand positions on any given day. You may not feel it, but your body learns each time you try.

Hold the Modified Headstand for 30 seconds.

When you can hold this position for 30 seconds comfortably, you are ready to go on. This could require a few days, weeks, or months. We are in no hurry.

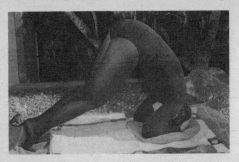

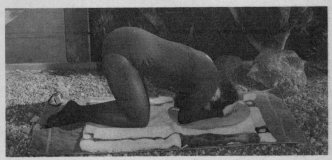

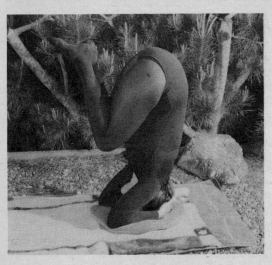

213

FIG. 185

In the slowest motion possible, begin to straighten your legs. This "halfway" position is a good stopping point. Don't go farther until you can hold this steadily for 30 seconds. There is no value in "shooting" the legs quickly upward from Fig. 184 to the completed position.

FIG. 186

Very slowly inch upward until the knees are straight. This is the Completed Headstand.

Eventually, we would want to be able to hold the body in an absolutely straight line, the legs aligned with the trunk as depicted. But this will take time. In the beginning simply attaining an approximate completed position is fine, and feeling quite unsteady so that you may not be able to maintain it for more than a few seconds is par for the course.

Come down the moment you feel your balance is becoming questionable. Rest a few moments with your head down as described in Fig. 183 and try once or twice more. We would like to avoid tumbling *forward,* so if you begin to lose your balance, keep the weight of your legs toward your chest and you will come down in the right direction.

The Modified Headstand and all positions intervening between the Modified and Completed postures can, in the beginning, make you somewhat dizzy or uncomfortably heavy in the upper extremities since, of course, the blood supply into these areas is increased quickly and directly. But here again the body seems to adjust to the inverted positions in a surprisingly short time so that in a few weeks all traces of any original discomfort disappear.

Begin with a 15 second hold in the completed posture, no longer. Attempt to add 5 seconds, no more, each time you do it. A hold of 3 to 5 minutes with absolute security will be our eventual goal. (As you become ready for the longer holds make sure to time yourself, so that your increase is *progressive;* don't do 15 seconds one day, 10 the next, 25 the next, 20 the next, and so forth. Once you add seconds you must be prepared to always hold for that number of seconds or minutes.)

In coming out of the completed posture we want to prevent the feet from "crashing" down to the floor. If you will simply reverse the way in which you straightened your legs upward, that is, bend your knees slowly and bring them close in toward your chest, you will be able to control the lowering movements.

When the toes touch the floor (lightly), lower your knees to the floor. Now move the legs back a few inches so that you can remain with your head down comfortably, relaxing all muscles for at least 30 seconds. Never raise your head immediately upon completion. Following the 30 second rest, very slowly raise your head and assume a seated posture (preferably the Lotus, described next).

I always advise those students who have high blood pressure, severe headaches, or a history of head or brain injury to obtain the approval of their physicians before doing the Headstand.

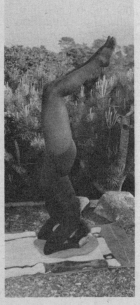
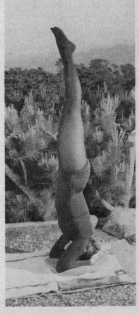

FULL-LOTUS

If you have been doing the "Arising" routine during the week, you are including two minutes of the cross-legged or Half-Lotus posture. In time (although we cannot predict how much time) the cross-legged posture can evolve into the Half-Lotus and the Half-Lotus into the Full-Lotus. If you have forgotten why these Lotus postures are important, reread the information on pp. 35.

During the past eleven years I have kept statistics in my Yoga classes and found that one out of every nine students can do the Full-Lotus in the first attempt; one out of every six students (who cannot do the Lotus in initial attempts) learns to do it within one to three months of practice. I know that a higher percentage learn to do it after the three month period but I have not kept records of this. Neither you or I can tell whether you will be successful in this posture; you can make no evaluation until you have practiced for a reasonable period because you cannot predict how supple your legs will become when subjected to the intensive stretching of these practices. But here again the practice itself is valuable for your legs. So in concluding our Weekend Routine with a few minutes of meditation, we can simultaneously attempt the Full-Lotus. Naturally, if this proves impossible, we simply revert to the Half-Lotus or cross-legged position.

FIG. 187

When you sit up from the Headstand, extend both legs straight outward.

Now take hold of your left foot and place it as high on the right thigh as possible. If your left knee will not rest on the floor at this point you cannot, at present, do the Full-Lotus. Simply rest your left forearm on your left leg and sit this way for a minute or two (while you are practicing meditation); then reverse the legs and rest the right forearm on the right leg for the second half of your meditation period. The weight of the arm will help to stretch your thigh so that the knee may eventually touch the floor. Once the knee is on the floor you can proceed to the final step that follows. However, if your knee is very far from the floor as you first attempt the Full-Lotus, you will probably feel a general discomfort and awkwardness that will not allow you to meditate properly. If this is the case you must revert to the Half-Lotus or cross-legged position until your legs gain in flexibility. Continue to attempt the Full-Lotus from time to time.

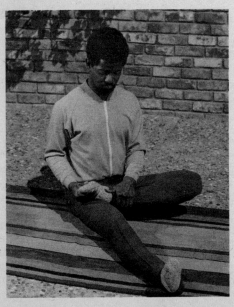

FIG. 188

This is the method of practice described above.

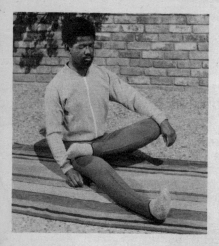

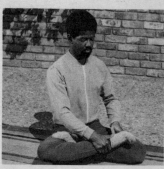

FIG. 189

Bring your right foot in toward you.

Take hold of it with your hands and place it on top of the left thigh. If discomfort is experienced, hold the position for only a few seconds (you can keep your hands on your right foot); then remove the right foot and stretch your legs outward.

If you can get into a Full-Lotus for only a few seconds you will very shortly be holding it for a minute or more. The legs adjust quickly.

FIG. 190

Here is the classical Full-Lotus with the *mudra* (hand and finger position) added. The index fingers touch the thumbs and the hands rest as illustrated. This position establishes "contact" of the subtle forces. The spine is erect but relaxed, the chin is aligned with the navel, the abdomen slightly protruded. Eyelids are lowered, not closed. This is the perfect posture for meditation.

Our model's right knee is slightly raised from his mat. He has been practicing the various Lotus positions for only four months and within another two months (or very possibly less) this knee will touch without difficulty. In the next photograph, where he is using two pillows, both knees rest on the mat easily.

Note the interesting triangular configuration of the body: the head is the apex, the legs the base, and imaginary lines from the head to the knees, the sides of the triangle. There are important esoteric *(tantrik)* implications of this triangle; primarily, the body derives increased life force from it, as it does from a number of geometric configurations. Many of the *asanas* you have learned from this book place the body in such configurations.

The moment your legs become tired, stretch them out. You can massage your knees or ankles with your hands if these areas are uncomfortable.

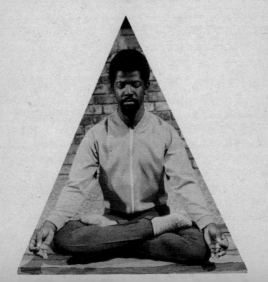

FIG. 191

Attempt the Full-Lotus with the legs reversed; because of the varying structure of the legs you may have more success on one side than on the other. Note that in this photograph our model is depicted sitting on two pillows. The raising of the buttocks automatically lowers the knees toward the floor. Try this and see if it is helpful but don't use the pillows if you don't need them.

Remember that we have no wish to torture your legs. You proceed, as in all Yoga postures, cautiously, in gradual stages. If you are successful, fine. If not, simply revert to an easier sitting position and continue to try the more advanced positions periodically. However, don't forget that the *practice* for the Full-Lotus will be of genuine value to your legs. They become supple, strengthened, firmed, and you will probably find that they regain a certain "spring," a youthful feeling.

As a final note I want to caution you against displaying the Lotus as an acrobatic accomplishment or a parlor trick. This posture is for the practice of private or group meditation and should be used only for this purpose. Neither the Lotus or Headstand, or, indeed, any of the *asanas* should ever be idly exhibited.

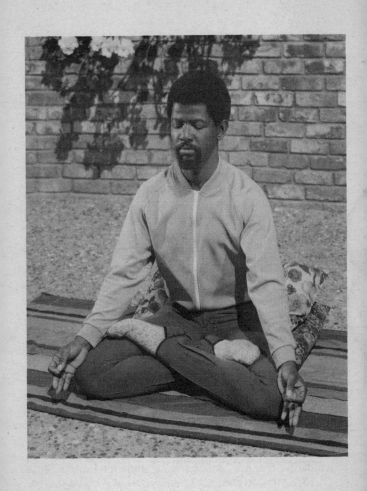

MEDITATION
(5–15 minutes)

We concluded our "Arising" routine with a brief meditation practice requiring approximately two minutes. Also, the conclusion of our "Before Retiring" routine called for two techniques—Alternate Nostril Breathing and Deep Relaxation—both of which can be considered meditation practices because of the profound state of tranquillity they induce. However, all three of these are *active* forms of meditation in the sense that we were actively involved in *doing* something: we chanted "OM," we breathed in a particular rhythm and pattern, we became acutely conscious of our bodies. Now I will ask you to conclude the Weekend Routine with a few minutes of the most profound type of meditation: *passive* meditation, that is, *doing absolutely nothing.*

Not infrequently the Yoga student decides that the exercises are fine and that he will devote serious efforts to perfecting them. But meditation—that's another matter. Meditation, he often feels, is something else, something removed, something beyond, something to do in later life when there will be more time. And it *is* possible to exclude meditation and still derive all of the benefits from the exercises that I have described. However, I must make it crystal clear that in the traditional practice of Yoga, meditation is an integral part of the study and cannot possibly be divorced from the physical movements. The *asanas* themselves are a form of *active* meditation (because of the manner in which your undivided attention is given to their performance), and *passive* meditation becomes the complementary half of the study. You must understand that, classically, the most important aspect of *Hatha* Yoga is that by removing tension, strengthening the nervous system, quieting the mind and emotions, arousing latent power, and cultivating a new awareness, it prepares

222

the organism for exactly this passive meditation. Therefore, if you are interested in the *total* Yoga practice, and if you are going to undertake the various routines in this book seriously, you will be in excellent physical and psychological condition to engage also in periods of meditation. We have practiced the active forms of meditation; now let us look at the passive.

First, it is important to list three things that passive meditation, in its Yogic context, is *not:* it is not prayer, it is not analysis, it is not a "trip." These represent a summary of the most common associations with the word "meditation," depending, of course, upon whom you are talking to. For many people "prayer" and "meditation" are interchangeable words. However, prayer is actually the articulation of a particular thought: it might be an expression of gratitude, it might be a request. This is not related to Yoga meditation. In the past decade in America exposure to the concepts of psychotherapy has become so widespread that more and more frequently I find people associating meditation with the practice of a type of introspection in which one involves himself in personality analysis, in examination of his "hang-ups," his good and bad points and, in general, in determining how he can derive more enjoyment from life. This is not related to Yoga meditation. Finally, due to a number of gross distortions and misinterpretations many young people have been led to believe that meditation is the vehicle through which it is possible to have a "blow-your-mind" experience, a sort of sound and light show, a fifth dimension "trip" similar to that which a drug might induce. Again, this has nothing to do with Yoga meditation. In passive Yoga meditation nothing is articulated to activate the mind or emotions, no analysis occurs to propagate the ego, no thrills or mystic experiences are sought to stimulate the nervous system. Passive meditation transcends all such concepts and its objectives are, in my opinion, the most profound that an individual can hope to attain: enlightenment and liberation. Achieving these constitutes the greatest adventure of life. But the foregoing phrases are deceiving unless they are read with a special eye because the "objective" is not understood nor the "adventure" undertaken in the way we usually conceive of such things. This is an "inner" adventure, and because it transpires passively in the most subtle recesses of one's being, it is comprised of a series of experiences, of stages of growth and expansion that cannot be accurately described. But you can begin this adventure *now* through passive meditation, the method of which is described below.

Having completed whatever physical routine you will perform, you now attempt to sit in the Half or Full-Lotus; if either of these is not yet possible, assume the simple cross-legged posture. Remember the hand, finger, and eye positions just described under Full-Lotus. Once you are comfortably settled, *become aware of your thoughts;* realize that you *are* thinking, that pictures and words are present in what we call the "mind." From where do these thoughts come? You don't know. To where do they go? Again, you don't know. You can give an intellectual answer that you may have learned; you can say, for example, "the subconscious," but you really know very little about this subconscious, and you do not actually perceive that this is where your thoughts come from and return to. So we know almost nothing about thoughts, how they are formed, where they come from, where they go to, why they appear when they do. And yet, while thoughts are present, while they occupy this "mind," they command our full attention; we identify wholly with these thoughts and actually consider them as "our thoughts." If there is one thing we almost never question it is the validity of our thoughts. As long as a thought is occupying the mind we believe it emanates from what we call "ourselves"; we reason that it must be a part of us and it must be there for some important purpose. Therefore, it deserves consideration, reflection, evaluation, action, dismissal, and so forth. But Yoga casts "thoughts" in a different light and offers a startling theory about the "mind." The essence of this theory is that we make an error of the greatest magnitude and create for ourselves the most horrendous "problems" by believing that the thoughts that arise are "ours," that they have arisen for a reason, and that they deserve our full attention until some disposition is made of them or until they simply disappear (only to be immediately replaced by another thought). Throughout our lives, almost every minute of our waking hours is spent in that process we call "thinking." A major aspect of what in Yoga is termed *maya* (illusion or ignorance) is related to the worshipping of, the devotion to our thoughts, when in reality most of what we identify as *our* thoughts have nothing to do with our true selves and actually result in a tragic waste of our time, of our lives.

Did you know you can stop thinking and that in the practice of Yoga it is of the greatest importance that you do just that periodically? When you learn how to switch off your mind you come to realize that most of your thinking is, indeed, a waste of invaluable time and energy. But most important of all, you come to understand, in the most profound sense of the word, that the *real* you, that spark of Universal Spirit that is responsible for your existence, lies behind the mind and that it is your constant preoccupation with thinking that obscures your knowledge and perception of your true spiritual nature. When you are able to quiet your mind, where there is a cessation of thoughts, you transcend your "ego," which only your thoughts have created and sustain. At that moment you are free, you know who you really are, you achieve "self-realization." You can never think, reason, debate, or analyze your way to enlightenment, freedom, and peace (*nirvana, samadhi,* the kingdom of heaven), but these lie always waiting to be *realized* the moment the illusion of a "self," an "ego" is dispelled by the cessation of thoughts. You have no *real* "self" and you have no *real* "mind"! If either of these were *real,* you could never experience true peace, enlightenment, and liberation.

We have now reached the point where nothing is to be gained by further exposition. What, from our usual viewpoint, we conceive of as the "mind" cannot, of course, envisage an existence without itself even for a moment, so all of the above discussion will only act to confuse you unless we have managed to reach that aspect of your intuitive wisdom that can recognize the necessity for turning off the thoughts. In this event we can proceed with our passive meditation method.

You have spent a few moments in observing your thoughts; you realize that you are thinking continually and that you have little or no conscious control of what comes into your mind. Now, find the "off" switch; *stop thinking;* discard all thoughts and perceptions. Remain in a state of nonthinking, of blankness. If thoughts arise cast them gently but firmly aside. It will be a revelation to you that thoughts can manifest themselves and that you can spend a surprising amount of time thinking about them and not be aware that you are thinking. That is, having decided you will not think, and desiring with your entire being not to think, you will, nonetheless, find yourself thinking! This is indicative of how your mind is constantly at work conjuring up words and pictures, from the sublime to the outrageous, and of how little control you have over the entire process. So you must be alert and aware of the arising of thoughts during your period of meditation and dismiss them as quickly as possible. You never become impatient or angry with your mind; you simply dismiss the thoughts gently but firmly and attempt to return to the "blank" state.

At first you may be able to maintain yourself in this void for only a few seconds at a time during the entire five minute period that I recommend to beginners for this practice. Gradually, however, just as we gain facility with all of the physical exercises through repeated attempts, the blank intervals increase in duration. When these intervals extend to several minutes, there is a transformation from a blank state to one of remarkable awareness and perception, the depth and intensity of which increase as you continue to meditate. No amount of description can convey what is experienced in this state. I have now told you everything you need to know at this time. Further guidance will be available to you as you require it; never be concerned about this. The essential thing is to begin your meditation *now* and allow nothing to interfere with regular practice.

Are one or two sessions during a weekend sufficient meditation for the week? Not really. Obviously, your progress is significantly accelerated if meditation is practiced on a daily basis, at the same hour each day, and for as much time as one can possibly devote. But the emphasis of this book is on complete practicality. I know you can probably devote the necessary time during the weekend, but that you may feel cramped for time if I suggest this practice daily, during the week. However, I also know that one always finds time to do what he really wants to do, and I believe that after a few weekends of meditating you will become profoundly cognizant of its value. Then you will begin to fit it into your week, usually meditating at the conclusion of the "Arising," or "Returning Home," or "Before Retiring" routines. As a beginning practice on weekends I suggest you devote five minutes to meditation. Approximate the five minutes without disturbing your meditation by continually glancing at a watch. I recommend five minutes because beginners tend to tire at about this point. But if you find the practice enjoyable, you can meditate for as long as you wish, even during first attempts. Extend your meditation time gradually so that you eventually work up to fifteen minutes. Many of my more advanced students spend as much as an hour or more in a single meditation session. The novice often thinks that this is a great deal of time to spend doing nothing. He has not yet realized that one's greatest growth, awareness, and power are cultivated in the type of inaction provided by deep meditation. When your legs tire in the cross-legged positions, either reverse them with as little movement and disturbance as possible or extend them straight outward and complete your meditation in this position. Remember, I told you that your ability to sit comfortably in the various Lotus postures will increase quickly and that these postures are definite aids in meditating.

In conclusion let me advise you not to look for results from your meditation sessions. This is peculiar advice because results are what we evaluate in any and all of our activities. We act so that certain results will ensue. (You will remember that in the "On the Job" section I wrote in a similar vein—not being "attached" to the fruits of your labor.) But meditation is not action, it is *inaction;* consequently, we cannot speak of the same type of results as we do with regard to action. The objectives here are different and results manifest themselves in what can be described as an "inverse" manner. For many months of meditation you will be in no position to evaluate your progress, so make no attempt to do so. You must simply continue to meditate regularly, attempting only to still your mind. There will come a time when you will suddenly be very much aware of a dramatic growth that has been occurring all the while!

For the present, all has been said. Essential aspects of the ancient sciences of *Hatha, Raja,* and *Karma* Yoga have been presented to you in a very palatable form; the routines and information in this book can be practically incorporated into your daily activities, no matter what they are. Now it's up to you.

THE ROUTINES AT A GLANCE

Once you are familiar with the various routines, these pages will provide ready reference charts to remind you of the order and repetitions of the exercises and approximately how much time should be spent with them. However, *continue to refer to the original instructions and illustrations of the exercises until you are absolutely certain you are doing each movement correctly.* Yoga offers great rewards in return for precision.

ARISING

Observation of Breathing (while still in bed) approx. 1:00

Breathing Routine	10 Charging Breaths followed by 1 Complete Breath, 5 times (See Fig. 5)	2:00
Leg Clasp	Your extreme position 3 times; hold for 10 each (See Fig. 8)	1:00
Rishi's Exercise	Your extreme position 3 times to each side, alternating sides; hold for 10 each (See Fig. 12)	2:00
Abdominal Lifts	Standing position: 3 groups of 10 movements All Fours position: 3 groups of 10 movements (See Fig. 17)	3:00
Meditation (in the Lotus)	The mantra "OM" 7 times (See Fig. 21)	2:00
		10:00

Chest Expansion	Backward bend; hold 5 Forward bend; hold 10 Stretch to each leg; hold 10 each Perform entire routine twice (See Fig. 28)	2:00
Head Twist	3 positions; hold 20 each Perform once (See Fig. 35)	1:00
Simple Spinal Twist	Your extreme position; hold 10 Twist twice to each side (See Fig. 40)	1:00
Back Stretch	One stretch with upper calves; hold 20 One stretch with lower calves or ankles; hold 20 (See Fig. 43)	1:00

5:00

Additional Exercises Optional

Dancer's Exercise	Continuous motion; 10 times (See Fig. 45)	2:00
Circular Motion	3 widening circles with trunk; hold each position for 2 Perform the complete 3 circle routine 5 times (See Fig. 54)	3:00

10:00

P.M. BREAK

Finger Exercise	Once with each finger Hold each stretch for 2 (See Fig. 55)	:15
Elbow Exercise	Perform 10 times in continuous motion (See Fig. 57)	:15
Shoulder Raise	Hold each raise for 5 Perform 3 times (See Fig. 60)	:30
Posture Clasp	Do the up and down pulls twice on each side Hold each pull for 5 (See Fig. 63)	1:00
Head Roll	4 positions; hold each for 5 Perform the entire routine 3 times in extremely slow motion (See Fig. 68)	1:15
Eye Exercise	4 positions; hold each for 1 Perform the entire routine 10 times Palm the eyes for approximately 30 (See Fig. 72)	1:15 :30

5:00

Additional Exercises Optional

Triangle	Perform twice below the knee on each side; alternate the sides Perform twice to the ankle area on each side; alternate the sides Hold each stretch for 10 (See Fig. 80)	2:30

231

Balance Posture	Perform 3 times on each side; alternate the sides Hold each stretch for 5 The variation, once on each side 2:30 (See Fig. 84)

10:00

RETURNING HOME

Back Stretch	Calves position, once; hold 20 Ankles position, once; hold 20 The extreme feet or toes position, once; hold 20 1:30 (See Fig. 91)
Bow	Moderate raise, once; hold 10 Extreme raise, once; hold 10 1:00 (See Fig. 96)
Alternate Leg Stretch	The following with each leg (the left first): calf position, once; hold 10 ankle position, once; hold 10 the extreme foot or toes position, once; hold 10 2:00 (See Fig. 103)
Knee and Thigh Stretch	Your extreme position, twice; hold 10 each :30 (See Fig. 107)

| Backward Bend | With feet on floor: moderate position, once; hold 10 extreme position, once; hold 10 With toes on floor: your extreme position, once; hold 10–20 | 1:00 |
| | (See Fig. 114) | |

| Shoulder Stand | Your extreme position, once; hold 1–5 minutes "Split," once; hold 10 Twists to left and right, once each; hold 10 each | average 3:00 |
| | (See Fig. 119) | |

| Breathing and Relaxation | Complete Breath, vigorous tapping with breath retained, followed by deep relaxation. Once. | approx. 1:00 |
| | (See Fig. 127) | |

10:00

BEFORE RETIRING

| Lion | 3 to 5 times; hold 20 each | 1:45 |
| | (See Fig. 129B) | |

| Scalp | In continuous motion: front area, 15 pulls back area, 15 pulls | :30 |
| | (See Fig. 130) | |

Chin and Throat Exercise	10 times; hold 2 each	:45
	(See Fig. 134)	
Cobra	Your extreme raise; hold 20 Twists to left and right, once each; hold 10 each Entire routine, twice (See Fig. 139)	2:30
Alternate Nostril Breathing	5 rounds in rhythms of 8–4–8. (Refer to the exercise for complete details) (See Fig. 143)	3:30
Deep Relaxation	Relaxing each area of the body by working slowly upward from the feet to the head Conclude with observation of breathing (See Fig. 146)	1:00

——————

10:00

WEEKEND PRACTICE

Perform this routine on one or both days of the weekend or whenever you wish to devote extra time to more intensive practice. Remember that you can also include as many other individual exercises or full routines as your time permits.

| Hip Bend | Moderate position to both sides; once each; hold 10 each Extreme position to both sides; twice each, alternating sides; hold 10 each (See Fig. 149) | 1:30 |

Full Twist	Your extreme twist to both sides, twice; hold 10 each (See Fig. 155B)	1:30
Side Raise	Left side: right leg, once; hold 10 both legs, moderate raise, once; hold 10 both legs, extreme raise, twice; hold 10 each Right side: identical (See Fig. 159)	2:00
Plough	Your extreme position of the 1st position; hold 20 When you can: 2nd position; hold 20 3rd position; hold 20 Your extreme Back Stretch position; hold 10 Perform the entire routine, twice (See Fig. 162)	3:00
Back Push-up	Extreme position, 3 times; hold 10 each Advanced position, once; hold 10 (See Fig. 171)	1:00
Locust	Left leg raise, once; hold 10 Right leg raise, once; hold 10 Both legs, moderate raise, once (with breath retained); hold 10 Your extreme raise (with breath retained) 3 times; hold 7 each (See Fig. 176)	2:00

| Headstand | Your extreme position, once (Refer to the exercise for all details regarding repetitions and holding times while you are in the learning process) (See Fig. 186) | Begin with as little as 5 seconds; with the addition of 5 second groups gradually work up to 3–5 minutes |
| Meditation (in the Half or Full-Lotus if possible) | Cessation of thoughts (See Fig. 190) | 5–15 minutes |

Average: 20–30 minutes

Mr. Hittleman's television series *Yoga For Health* may be seen in many areas. For a free Newsletter and catalogue of the author's record albums, write to:

Richard Hittleman
Carmel Valley, California, 93924

DO MORE FOR YOUR HEALTH WITH THESE GREAT BOOKS FROM WARNER PAPERBACK LIBRARY!

_____ **SLIMMING DOWN**
by Ed McMahon (78-118, $1.50)

_____ **YOGA FOR BEAUTY AND HEALTH** by Eugene Rawls and Eve Diskin (78-493, $1.50)

_____ **BE YOUNG WITH YOGA**
by Richard L. Hittleman (76-419, $1.25)

_____ **RENEW YOUR LIFE THROUGH YOGA**
by Indra Devi (66-932, $1.25)

_____ **THERE IS A CURE FOR THE COMMON COLD** by Edme Regnier, M.D. (66-984, $1.25)

_____ **THE STRAIGHT STORY ON V.D.** by Hans H. Neumann, M.D. with Sylvia Simmons
(76-354, $1.25)

_____ **MARTINIS AND WHIPPED CREAM** by Sidney Petrie in association with Robert B. Stone
(65-017, 95¢)

_____ **YOGA FOR PHYSICAL FITNESS** by Richard L. Hittleman (76-601, $1.25)

W A Warner Communications Company

If you are unable to obtain these books from your local dealer, they may be ordered directly from the publisher.

Please allow 4 weeks for delivery.

WARNER PAPERBACK LIBRARY
P.O. Box 690
New York, N.Y. 10019

Please send the books I have checked.

I am enclosing payment plus 15¢ per copy to cover postage and handling. New York State residents add applicable sales tax.

Name ....

Address ....

City .... State .... Zip ....

_____ Please send me your free mail order catalog